NUTRITION,
the AGED,
and SOCIETY

Cary S. Kart
Seamus P. Metress
University of Toledo

NUTRITION, the AGED, and SOCIETY

PRENTICE-HALL, INC., Englewood Cliffs, New Jersey 07632

Library of Congress Cataloging in Publication Data

KART, CARY STEVEN.
  Nutrition, the aged, and society.

  Includes bibliographies and index.
    1. Aging—Nutritional aspects.   2. Aged—Nutrition.
  3. Nutrition policy—United States.   I. Metress,
  Seamus P.   II. Title. [DNLM: 1. Aged—United States.
  2. Geriatrics.   3. Nutrition—In old age.   WT 100 Kl8n]
  QP86.K38 1984   362.1'76   83-4531
  ISBN 0-13-627521-4

Editorial/production supervision: *Edith Riker*
Manufacturing buyer: *Harry Baisley*
Cover design: *Wanda Lubelska Design*

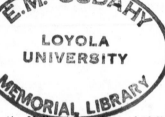

Printed in the United States of America
10 9 8 7 6 5 4 3 2 1

ISBN 0-13-627521-4

Prentice-Hall International, Inc., *London*
Prentice-Hall of Australia Pty. Limited, *Sydney*
Editora Prentice-Hall do Brasil, Ltda., *Rio de Janiero*
Prentice-Hall Canada Inc., *Toronto*
Prentice-Hall of India Private Limited, *New Delhi*
Prentice-Hall of Japan, Inc., *Tokyo*
Prentice-Hall of Southeast Asia Pte. Ltd., *Singapore*
Whitehall Books Limited, *Wellington, New Zealand*

CONTENTS

PREFACE

The study of aging varies in its focus. Gerontologists, who systematically study aging, say it is a multidisciplinary undertaking because the major elements of the field are drawn from a number of physical and social sciences. However, this multidisciplinary tag also reflects an identity crisis in the field. A joint study committee of the Association for Gerontology in Higher Education and the Gerontological Society of America has found that little consensus exists about the common core of knowledge in gerontology. Defining consensus as 90 percent agreement, this committee found that gerontological educators and practitioners could agree on only three topics for inclusion in the content of gerontology—the biology of aging, the psychology of aging, and health and aging. Other topics that came close to receiving a consensus vote included demography of aging, sensory change, the sociology of aging, and environment and aging.

Noticeably absent from this list is the topic of nutrition and aging. Yet we believe that it deserves status in the enterprise of gerontology. While our own interest in this topic is a natural extension of earlier work done in connection with health and aging, nutrition clearly is relevant to other topical areas in gerontology. In part, we have learned on our own about the relevance of nutrition to these other areas (for example, biology, psychology), but we have also been taught about this relevance by the students in our gerontology classes. These students represent a great diversity of professional interests—nursing, medicine, and dentistry; health education and the allied health professions; sociology and social work, anthropology, psychology and home economics. It is for these students of aging that we have prepared this primer.

This book will serve as an introduction to the role of nutrition in the aging process. Several of the major theories of biological aging include nutrition as one mechanism which appears to be involved in the complex process of aging. Nutrition also plays an important part in the course of many degenerative diseases. Additionally, food may be as important to the elderly for social-psychological reasons as it is for physiological well-being.

Chapter 1 presents an overview of the biological theories of aging. Chapter 2 demographically profiles the elderly population of the U.S. National, regional and local studies of the nutritional status of the aged are summarized in Chapter 3. Chapters 4 and 5 discuss the nutritional needs of older people as well as the biocultural basis of geriatric nutrition. Chapter 6 looks at the relationship of nutrition to aging and disease. Society's programmatic response to the nutritional problems of the elderly is covered in Chapter 7 while the Epilogue considers the likelihood of a national nutrition policy. Chapters 1, 2, 3, 7, and the Epilogue were written by Cary Kart; Chapters 4, 5, and 6 by Seamus Metress.

Special acknowledgements go to Carol Engler and Marye Shinn for their editorial assistance and to Angie Christensen, Jan Fogel, and Marjorie Managhan for the typing. Thanks go as well to several anonymous reviewers who made helpful substantive and stylistic comments. Finally, our editors at Prentice-Hall, and especially Edie Riker, deserve a special commendation for helping to bring this project to fruition.

CHAPTER ONE
THE AGING PROCESS

If one believes Homer, Sisyphus was the wisest and most prudent of mortals (Camus, 1955). Supposedly, he even outsmarted the gods and held off the inevitability of his own death. Being near to death, Sisyphus instructed his wife to omit the appropriate funerary sacrifices and to cast his unburied body into the middle of the public square. He awoke in the underworld and, after expressing mock indignation at his wife's failure to carry out the funerary rituals, received permission from Pluto to return to earth—and to life—in order to reprimand his wife. Camus (1955) wrote, "Many years more he lived facing the curve of the gulf, the sparkling sea, and the smiles of earth." Ultimately, as the myth goes, a decree of the gods was necessary to return Sisyphus to the underworld, for even he had to suffer this inevitable result of old age.

For some, Sisyphus personifies a belief in the desirability of attempting to hold off death in order to lengthen life. This is a prominent motif that is evident in past and present writings about aging and death (Gruman, 1966). Three different themes recur in these writings concerning the search for the means of prolonging life. The *antedeluvian theme* involves the belief that people lived much longer in the past. This theme is best exemplified in the book of Genesis, which records the life spans of ten Hebrew partriarchs who lived before the flood. Among them are Noah, who lived for 950 years, and

Methuselah, who survived for 969 years. Second, the *hyperborean theme* involves the idea that in some remote part of the world there are people who enjoy a remarkably long life. According to the traditions of ancient Greece, a certain people lived *hyper Boreas* (beyond the north wind):

> Their hair crowned with golden bay-leaves they hold glad revelry; and neither sickness nor baneful eld mingleth among the chosen people; but, aloof from toil and conflict, they dwell afar (Gruman, 1966:22).

The third, or *fountain theme*, is based on the idea that some unusual substance exists which has the property of greatly increasing the length of life (Gruman, 1966). The search for the "fountain of youth" by Juan Ponce de Leon, who accidently discovered Florida in 1513, is a good example of this rejuvenation theme. According to the earliest account of Ponce de Leon's adventure, published by a Spanish official in the New World in 1535, the explorer was "seeking that fountain of Biminie that the Indians had given to be understood would renovate or resprout and refresh the age and forces of he who drank or bathed himself in that fountain" (Lawson, 1946 in Gruman, 1966).

These themes retain their relevance in the present. Interestingly, each has also been employed in a way that suggests a positive relationship exists between nutrition and longevity. For example, to some, the antedeluvian theme highlights the need to return to food consumption patterns of the distant past. After all, Methuselah consumed neither "junk food" nor food containing additives or colorings and he supposedly lived to be 969 years old. We can only guess that the Hebrew patriarch ate "natural" foods since what we know about food storage techniques and facilities available before the flood suggests that everything he ate was fresh. Perhaps the Hebrew patriarchs were also "fathers" of the current natural foods movement so popular in some nutrition circles today.

Our fascination with the reportedly "long-lived" Abkhasians of the Georgian Republic of Russia reflects a modern-day hyperborean theme. The Abkhasians attribute their longevity to particular practices in relation to sex, work and diet (Benet, 1971). For instance, their diet is quite stable. They show few idiosyncratic preferences and do not significantly change their food consumption patterns throughout the course of their lives. According to anthropologist Sula Benet (1971, 1974), their caloric intake is about one-fourth lower than that of comparable industrial workers in the same region of the Soviet Union, though they consume twice as much vitamin C. The Abkhasians eat very little meat or fish. Dietary staples include fresh fruits and vegetables as well as *abista*, a corn meal mash cooked in water without salt that takes the place of bread. Few Abkhasians smoke; they drink neither coffee nor tea, but adults, on the average, consume two glasses of buttermilk a day in addition to small quantities of a locally produced dry red wine of low alcoholic content (Benet, 1971). Sugar is conspicuously absent from their diet.

Soviet medical authorities believe that the local diet adds years to the lives of the Abkhasians. In particular, they speculate that the buttermilk, pickled vegetables, and probably the wine help destroy certain bacteria, which may indirectly prevent the development of arteriosclerosis. Unfortunately, there are many reasons for doubting the validity of claims that groups such as the Abkhasians have a statistically high proportion of centenarians in their population (Kyncharyants, 1974; Medvedev, 1974, 1975). The Russian gerontologist Medvedev contends that none of these supposed cases of superlongevity is scientifically valid. He believes that many "long-lived" Georgians are, in fact, army deserters from the First World War who forged documents or used their fathers' in order to escape remobilization.

Finally, any student of American billboard and television advertising will recognize the fountain theme. A plethora of different foods and vitamins, as well as skin creams hair colorings, and body soaps, are all depicted as unusual substances that we may use to remain eternally young. However, while some of these substances (vitamins C and E, for example) have been employed to successfully extend the lives of experimental laboratory animals, considerably more research is needed to understand the potential applications of specific substances in deterring the aging process in humans.

The perenniality of these three themes suggests that throughout history up until the present, people have had difficulty distinguishing between myth and history and between magic and science. The development of the as yet "unfinished" sciences of nutrition and gerontology can be seen in this light. Both nutrition, the science that deals with the effects of food on the body (Mayer, 1974), and gerontology, the systematic study of the aging process, reflect organized attempts to make clear distinctions between myth and history, magic and science.

The fields of nutrition and gerontology have at least three points of intersection. Identifying these intersections is important because they set the parameters of the emerging field of geriatric nutrition. First, there is a growing belief that nutrition plays a part in biological aging, though most of the data supporting this contention is open to debate. Essentially, the role of nutrition in biological aging remains undefined. Second, nutritional scientists, health care professionals, and even the general public have an increasing awareness of the relationship between nutrition and disease. It is common knowledge, for instance, that the elderly are at higher risk than the young for developing certain chronic diseases including heart disease, cancer, cerebrovascular disease, hypertension and arthritis. A current, well-developed literature describes the role of certain dietary elements in preventing or improving, or causing or exacerbating particular disease states. Already, conclusions drawn from this research are being converted into clinical care regimens intended to reduce the incidence of some of these disorders as well as their impact on elderly individuals who contract them. Finally, we are coming to understand the relationship between the social aspects of aging and nutrition. Aging does *not* occur in a psychosocial vacuum. For example, many of the elderly are subject to multiple role changes, which may be brought on by retirement, widowhood and dependency, and which can have significant impact on their nutritional status and health. Clearly, health professionals must recognize these nonphysiological factors when evaluating the nutritional status of elderly clients.

MORTALITY AND LIFE EXPECTANCY AMONG THE ELDERLY

When do we become old? At what age does our vulnerability increase to a level at which it becomes a real threat to life? These are difficult questions. Aging is, after all, a real biological process and some of us show our vulnerability to it early in life. Gerontologists use the term *senescence* to describe this increasing vulnerability. Put more formally, senescence is a general term used to describe the group of effects that lead to a decreasing expectation of life with increasing age (Comfort, 1979). Strehler (1962) distinguishes senescence from other biological processes in four ways: (1) its characteristics are universal; (2) the changes which constitute it come from within the individual; (3) the processes associated with senescence occur gradually; and (4) the changes which appear in senescence have a negative effect on the individual. Yet Comfort (1979) doubts that senescence is " . . . a 'fundamental,' 'inherent,' or otherwise generalizable process." Further, he believes that attempts to identify a single underlying property that explains all instances of senescent change are misplaced.

However, there still appears to be some pattern to our increased vulnerability through the life course. Table 1.1 presents death rates by color, sex and age for the United States in 1977. As the table indicates, men and women of all races die at all ages, though at varying rates which increase exponentially through the life cycle. Roughly speaking, it appears that the probability of dying doubles every eight years. While we can accept the principle that the probability of dying increases with age, it is important to emphasize that the probabilities themselves differ for males and females and differ also according to race, among other variables, and change over time.

Sex and Mortality

As can be seen from Table 1.1, comparisons by race show that men have higher death rates than women in every age category. Some of this difference in mortality rate is almost certainly attributable to biological factors. The larger proportion of males who die in infancy is not otherwise easily explainable by factors such as systematic variation in physical and/or social environment. For adults, though, it is difficult to distinguish biological from environ-

TABLE 1.1. Death rates for all causes, according to race, sex and age: United States, 1977.[1] (Data are based on the national vital registration system; Number of deaths per 100,000 resident population.)

	TOTAL[2]	WHITE MALE	WHITE FEMALE	BLACK MALE	BLACK FEMALE
All ages, crude	878.1	998.2	783.3	1,037.0	730.6
All ages, age adjusted[3]	612.3	781.5	427.8	1,127.6	664.4
Under 1 year	1,485.6	1,429.7	1,094.8	3,038.7	2,509.6
1–4 years	68.8	69.7	55.0	113.6	91.0
5–9 years	34.0	38.4	25.6	53.6	35.6
10–14 years	35.1	42.5	25.0	55.7	28.3
15–19 years	101.6	145.8	55.2	143.0	62.0
20–24 years	133.5	190.0	59.3	287.2	102.7
25–29 years	132.1	167.3	61.4	412.8	143.8
30–34 years	140.9	164.2	78.3	465.8	178.2
35–39 years	195.5	219.3	115.6	610.0	275.8
40–44 years	304.7	339.7	191.7	862.9	440.6
45–49 years	482.3	565.1	309.7	1,206.2	658.4
50–54 years	754.7	925.4	480.1	1,765.1	998.5
55–59 years	1,138.1	1,440.0	726.2	2,472.3	1,397.3
60–64 years	1,784.9	2,338.0	1,144.0	3,565.0	1,987.4
65–69 years	2,480.4	3,436.4	1,632.7	3,937.4	2,234.5
70–74 years	3,847.1	5,233.9	2,634.6	6,699.0	4,606.8
75–79 years	6,073.0	8,104.6	4,603.3	9,886.7	7,271.0
80–84 years	8,814.7	11,597.5	7,494.9	9,853.8	6,618.5
85 years and over	14,725.9	18,041.7	14,039.7	12,030.0	9,035.3

[1] Excludes deaths of nonresidents of the United States.
[2] Includes all races and both sexes.
[3] Age adjusted by the direct method to the total population of the United States as enumerated in 1940, using 11 age groups.
Source: U.S. Department of Health and Human Services, *Health, United States, 1980.* DHHS Publication No. (PHS) 81-1232, Table 8, pp. 127–130, Washington, D.C., U.S. Government Printing Office, December, 1980.

mental influences. The childbearing experience of females as well as the over-representation of males in dangerous occupations are examples of factors which make it difficult to quantify the relative effect on mortality of biological and environmental or sociocultural factors.

One attempt at differentiating biological from environmental factors in mortality was carried out by Francis Madigan (1957). In this study he compared the mortality rates of Catholic brothers and nuns who were members of teaching communities. Madigan argued that the life experiences of these two groups were quite similar—that is, brothers and nuns were subjected to the same sociocultural strains and stresses. Of particular importance here was the absence of sex-linked activities relevant to mortality—childbearing for females and participation in dangerous occupations for males. Madigan found that the difference in mortality rates between brothers and nuns was greater than between males and females in the population as a whole. This difference had been increasing during the decades under study. From the data obtained, he concluded that biological factors are more important than sociocultural ones. He hypothesized that, under conditions of equal stress, women were no more resistant to infections and contagious diseases than men, but had a greater constitutional resistance to degenerative diseases.

Such a hypothesis is difficult to test empirically. Table 1.2 presents ratios of male to female death rates for the population 55 years of age and over, by age, from 1900 to 1976. In general, the table shows increasing male-female mortality differences throughout this century that very likely reflect a major shift in the cause-pattern of mortality. During the twentieth century, the contribution of infectious and parasitic diseases and maternal mortality to overall mortality rates has diminished relative to that of the chronic degenerative diseases such as diseases of the heart, malignant neoplasms, and cerebrovascular diseases (Seigel, 1979). However, changes in recent decades in the male-female mortality ratio appear to be more associated with social and environmental factors than biological ones. For example, according to Petersen (1975), the age-adjusted death rate from cancers was 65 *percent higher for females* than males in 1900, about equal between the sexes in 1947, and *20 percent higher for males* by 1963. This changing pattern probably has more to do with technological advancements than innate biological factors. For instance, the diagnosis and cure of cancers most frequent among females, breast and uterine, has improved at a more rapid rate than cancers most frequent among males, those of the lung and digestive system. Changes in social behavior may also foretell changes in the male-female mortality ratio. For example, recent slower rates of increase in male mortality are attributed, in part, to lowered smoking rates while, according to the American Cancer Society (1978), the increase in smoking among women may eventually cause female lung cancer deaths to outnumber breast cancer deaths by the mid-1980s.

TABLE 1.2.   Ratios of male-to-female death rates for the population 55 years old and over, by age: U.S., 1900 to 1976.

YEAR	55 TO 64 YEARS	65 TO 74 YEARS	74 TO 84 YEARS	85 YEARS AND OVER	65 YEARS AND OVER
1900	1.14	1.11	1.08	1.05	1.06
1940	1.45	1.29	1.17	1.08	1.17
1954	1.82	1.57	1.29	1.06	1.30
1968	2.07	1.88	1.46	1.18	1.44
1976	1.99	1.97	1.58	1.26	1.46

Source: Siegel, Jacob S. *Prospective Trends in the Size and Structure of the Elderly Population, Impact of Mortality Trends, and Some Implications.* CPR, Special Studies Series P-23 No. 78, Table 7. U.S. Department of Commerce, Bureau of the Census: Washington, D.C., U.S. Government Printing Office.

As a final comment on the Madigan study, it should be noted that many mortality-related factors which could have accounted for the difference in death rates between brothers and nuns were not taken into account—two examples are smoking behavior and obesity.

Race and Mortality

The large disparity in mortality rates that appears when comparing members of different racial groups does not often receive the attention it deserves because it is a hidden factor. If we return to Table 1.1 and look across the first row labeled "all ages, crude," it can be observed that the death rate of black males is slightly higher than that of white males (1037.0 v. 998.2) while the death rate for black females is *slightly lower* than that for white females (730.6 v. 783.3). However, because of higher birthrates, blacks have a younger age structure, which tends to mask true mortality. If we examine mortality across the second row, "all ages, age-adjusted," and in individual age groups, the full impact of race on mortality emerges. For example, infant mortality in the U.S. in 1977 was 129 percent higher among black than white females (2509.6 v. 1094.8) and 113 percent higher among black than white males. Death rates among young adults 25-59 years of age is 147 percent greater for black males (412.8 v. 167.3) and 134 percent greater for black females (143.8 v. 61.4) than for their white counterparts. It is only at age eighty that this racial differential in death rates disappears. None of this comes as a great surprise to demographer Donald Bogue (1969:595-6): "Throughout almost all of the ages when great progress in death control has been accomplished, death rates for [blacks] are about double those of whites."

While there has been some long-term progress in reducing the racial differences in mortality, this has slowed recently. In 1900, the age-adjusted death rates for nonwhites was 58 percent higher than the comparable figures for whites; in 1965 this differential was 45 percent and by 1975 it was 39 percent. The race differential in mortality is greater for females than for males. As Table 1.1 shows, black males had an age-adjusted death rate which was 44 percent higher (1127.6 v. 781.5) than the rate for white males in 1977; this differential for females was 55 percent (664.4 v. 427.8). Also, the sex differential in mortality is smaller for blacks than for the white population. In general, it appears that nonwhite women have been able to take less advantage of available technological advancements in death control than have nonwhite men (Bogue, 1969; 596-7).

Two additional points need be stressed when dealing with racial differentials in mortality. First, there is no reason to believe that blacks in particular and nonwhites in general are less biologically fit than whites in their capacity to survive. This point emphasizes that racial differentials in mortality reflect unnecessarily high mortality among nonwhites. Secondly, other factors, not the least of which is socioeconomic status, confound mortality data. Kitagawa and Hauser (1973) have shown the age-adjusted mortality rates for Japanese-Americans to be about one-third the corresponding rates for whites and one-half as large as the rate for blacks. Their additional analysis of median family income among these groups suggests that socioeconomic status may account for a considerable proportion of the race differentials in mortality. This is depicted in the figure below, which shows the inverse relationship between median family income and mortality.

RANK ORDER IN TERMS OF MEDIAN FAMILY INCOME (HIGHEST TO LOWEST)	RANK ORDER IN TERMS OF AGE-ADJUSTED MORTALITY RATES (HIGHEST TO LOWEST)
Japanese	Black
White	White
Black	Japanese

How does low socioeconomic status contribute to the higher mortality rates prevalent among blacks? Their lack of access to high quality medical care is one reason. According to the U.S. Office of Health Resources (1979), black people receive considerably fewer preventive services, on the average, than do white people. Also, treatment of blacks is often delayed until the onset of later stages of disease. (Gonnella, Louis and McCord, 1976).

While we are unable to say precisely whether biological or social factors are more important contributors to mortality differentials among different population groups in our society, it should be clear that biological aging does not occur in a social vacuum. Age-adjusted death rates in our total population are, for example, only about one-third of what they were at the beginning of this century. Additionally, even when considering those who, as a group, are already chronologically old (65 years of age and older), there has been a significant decline (27 percent) in death rates since 1950 (see Table 1.3). These reductions in the overall death rates of our population reflect at least four factors, all of which involve attempts begun in the nineteenth century to increase control over the environment (Dorn, 1959): (1) increased food supply; (2) development of commerce and transportation; (3) changes in technology and industry; and (4) increased control over infectious disease.

Progress in the reduction of mortality is also reflected in figures for average life expectancy at birth. Average life expectancy at birth, defined as the average number of years a person born today can expect to live under current mortality conditions, has shown great improvement in this century. This figure rose from 47.3 years in 1900 to 69.7 years in 1960 and 73.2 years in 1977 Table 1.4). This change constitutes a 55 percent increase in life expectancy at birth in three-quarters of a century, or an average annual gain in life expectancy of approximately one-third of a year during each year of this period. Still, just as there are significant sex and racial differentials in mor-

TABLE 1.3. Age-adjusted death rates for selected causes of death: United States, selected years 1950-77.[1] (Data are based on the national vital registration system.)

CAUSE OF DEATH	1950	1955	1960	1965	1970	1975	1976	1977
				YEAR				
	Deaths per 100,000 resident population							
All causes	841.5	764.5	760.9	739.0	714.3	638.3	627.5	612.3
Diseases of the heart	307.6	287.5	286.2	273.9	253.6	220.5	216.7	210.4
Cerebrovascular disease	88.8	83.0	79.7	72.7	66.3	54.5	51.4	48.2
Malignant neoplasms	125.4	125.8	125.8	127.0	129.9	130.9	132.3	133.0
Respiratory system	12.8	16.0	19.2	23.0	28.4	32.5	33.5	34.3
Digestive system	47.7	43.5	41.1	38.3	35.2	33.6	33.6	33.4
Breast[2]	22.2	22.7	22.3	22.8	23.1	22.8	23.1	23.5
Influenza and pneumonia	26.2	21.0	28.0	23.5	22.1	16.6	17.4	14.2
Bronchitis, emphysema, and asthma	—	—	—	—	11.6	8.6	7.9	7.2
Tuberculosis	21.7	8.4	5.4	3.6	2.2	1.2	1.1	1.0
Cirrhosis of liver	8.5	9.4	10.5	12.1	14.7	13.8	13.6	13.1
Diabetes mellitus	14.3	13.0	13.6	13.4	14.1	11.6	11.1	10.4
All accidents	57.5	54.4	49.9	53.3	53.7	44.8	43.2	43.8
Motor vehicle accidents	23.3	24.6	22.5	26.5	27.4	21.3	21.5	22.4
Suicide	11.0	9.9	10.6	11.4	11.8	12.6	12.3	12.9
Homicide	5.4	4.8	5.2	6.2	9.1	10.5	9.5	9.6

[1]Age-adjusted rates are computed by the direct method to the total population of the United States as enumerated in 1940, using 11 age groups.
[2]Female only.

Source: National Center for Health Statistics: Vital Statistics Rates in the United States, 1940–1960, by R. D. Grove and A.M. Hetzel. DHEW Pub. No. (PHS) 1677. Public Health Service. Washington. U.S. Government Printing Office, 1968; Unpublished data from the Division of Vital Statistics.

TABLE 1.4. Life expectancy at birth and at 65 years of age, according to color and sex: United States, selected years 1900–1977. (Data are based on the national vital registration system.)

SPECIFIED AGE AND YEAR	TOTAL			WHITE			ALL OTHER		
	BOTH SEXES	MALE	FEMALE	BOTH SEXES	MALE	FEMALE	BOTH SEXES	MALE	FEMALE
At birth			Remaining life expectancy in years						
1900[1]	47.3	46.3	48.3	47.6	46.6	48.7	33.0	32.5	33.5
1950	68.2	65.6	71.1	69.1	66.5	72.2	60.8	59.1	62.9
1960	69.7	66.6	73.1	70.6	67.4	74.1	63.6	61.1	66.3
1970[2]	70.9	67.1	74.8	71.7	68.0	75.6	65.3	61.3	69.4
1975[2]	72.5	68.7	76.5	73.2	69.4	77.2	67.9	63.6	72.3
1976[2]	72.8	69.0	76.7	73.5	69.7	77.3	68.3	64.1	72.6
1977[2]	73.2	69.3	77.1	73.8	70.0	77.7	68.8	64.6	73.1
At 65 years									
1900-1902[1]	11.9	11.5	12.2	—	11.5	12.2	—	10.4	11.4
1950	13.9	12.8	15.0	—	12.8	15.1	—	12.5	14.5
1960	14.3	12.8	15.8	14.4	12.9	15.9	13.9	12.7	15.2
1970[2]	15.2	13.1	17.0	15.2	13.1	17.1	14.9	13.3	16.4
1975[2]	16.0	13.7	18.0	16.0	13.7	18.1	15.7	13.7	17.5
1976[2]	16.0	13.7	18.0	16.1	13.7	18.1	15.8	13.8	17.6
1977[2]	16.3	13.9	18.3	16.3	13.9	18.4	16.0	14.0	17.8

[1]Death registration area only. The death registration area increased from 10 States and the District of Columbia in 1900 to the coterminous United States in 1933.

[2]Excludes deaths of nonresidents of the United States.

Source: National Center for Health Statistics: Vital Statistics Rates in the United States 1940–1960 by R.D. Grove and A.M. Hetzel. DHEW Pub. No. (PHS) 1977. Public Health Service. Washington. U.S. Government Printing Office, 1968; Vital Statistics of the United States, 1970, Vol. II, Part A. DHEW Pub. No. (HRA) 75–1101. Health Resources Administration. Washington. U.S. Government Printing Office, 1974; Final mortality statistics, 1975–1977. Monthly Vital Statistics Report Vols. 25, 26, and 28, Nos. 11, 12, and 1. DHEW Pub. Nos. (HRA) 77–1120, (PHS) 78–1120, and (PHS) 79–1120. Health Resources Administration and Public Health Service. Washington. U.S. Government Printing Office, Feb. 11, 1977, Mar. 30, 1978, and May 11, 1979; Unpublished data from the Division of Vital Statistics.

tality, there are similar differentials in life expectancy. As Table 1.4 shows us, the population group with the highest life expectancy at birth in 1977 is white females (77.7 years); nonwhite males have the lowest life expectancy (64.6 years). All groups have substantially increased life expectancy compared to that seen in 1900. The introduction of better sanitary conditions, the development of effective public health programs, and an increased standard of living are three additional factors often cited with those listed above to explain increased life expectancy in this century.

Life expectancy at birth is a function of death rates at all ages. Thus this statistic does not tell us at what specific ages improvement has occurred. We are particularly interested in judging progress in "survivorship" for those 65 and over. One technique for summarizing such changes in survivorship is to look to *life table* survival rates. A life table shows what the probability is of surviving from one age to any subsequent age based on the age-specific death rates at a particular time and place (Petersen, 1975). According to the life table for 1900–02, 39 percent of the newborn babies would reach age 65

TABLE 1.5.   Abridged life table for the total population: United States, 1970.

AGE INTERVAL	PROPORTION DYING	OF 100,000 BORN ALIVE	
PERIOD OF LIFE BETWEEN TWO EXACT AGES STATED IN YEARS	PROPORTION OF PERSONS ALIVE AT BEGINNING OF AGE INTERVAL DYING DURING INTERVAL	NUMBER LIVING AT BEGINNING OF AGE INTERVAL	NUMBER DYING DURING AGE INTERVAL
(1)	(2)	(3)	(4)
0–1	0.0202	100,000	2,016
1–5	.0034	97,984	331
5–10	.0021	97,653	205
10–15	.0020	97,448	198
15–20	.0055	97,250	535
20–25	.0074	97,715	713
25–30	.0072	96,002	690
30–35	.0086	95,312	821
35–40	.0123	94,491	1,161
40–45	.0187	93,330	1,745
45–50	.0288	91,585	2,640
50–55	.0436	88,945	3,876
55–60	.0660	85,069	5,611
60–65	.0956	79,458	7,600
65–70	.1386	71,858	9,960
70–75	.1976	61,989	12,234
75–80	.2885	49,664	14,330
80–85	.4035	35,334	14,257
85 and over	1.0000	21,077	21,077

Source: U.S. Public Health Service. Vital Statistics of the United States, 1970, Vol. 2, Section 5: Life Tables. Washington, D.C., 1973. Table 5.1.

whereas the life table of 1970 indicates that that figure would be almost 72 percent (see Table 1.5, column 3). The proportion of persons surviving from age 65 to age 80 was 33 percent in 1900–02 and about 50 percent in 1970—a gain of 17 persons reaching age 80 per 100 persons aged 65.

Another technique for measuring changes in survivorship involves looking at changes in age-specific life expectancy. Table 1.4 presents life expectancies at birth and age 65 by sex and race in the United States for selected years. Life expectancy at age 65 has moved ahead more slowly than life expectancy at birth since 1900. The small increase (4.4 years) of "expectation" values for those 65 and over between 1900 and 1977 is in part a function of the relative lack of success the medical sciences have had in reducing adult deaths caused by heart disease, cancer and cerebrovascular diseases. These have been the leading causes of death among persons 65 years and over since 1950. While some progress has been made in reducing death rates due to heart disease and cerebrovascular diseases in the last quarter of a century, the death rate from malignant neoplasms (cancer) has increased by more than 12 percent since 1950.

When do we become old? This is difficult to say with any precision. Gerontologists continue to argue over the relative efficiency of chronological or symptomatic definitions of old age. However, based on the above discussion of progress made in the reduction of death rates and increases in life expectancy, it still appears that, in general, we become vulnerable to old age later in the life span than those who came before us. Those who follow us will, in turn, probably be susceptible to old age at an even more chronologically advanced point in the life span.

BIOLOGICAL THEORIES
OF AGING

Why do we become old?[1] Answers to this question have been offered at both the cellular and physiological levels. According to Comfort (1979), there are four classical hypotheses that attempt to explain the mechanism of aging. These include the beliefs that vigor declines (1) through changes in the properties of multiplying cells; (2) through loss of, or injury to, non-multiplying cells (for example, neurons); and (3) through primary changes in the noncellular materials of the body (for example, collagen). A fourth hypothesis locates the mechanism of aging in the "software" of the body—"in the overall program of regulation by which other aspects of the life cycle are governed" (Comfort, 1979:17). These hypotheses are not necessarily mutually exclusive. As Comfort has pointed out, though some of these hypotheses have been around for several hundred years, none has yet been eliminated by convincing experimental data. The alert reader may recognize these classic hypotheses in the following brief summaries of research in biological aging.

[1]This section borrows heavily from Baker and Allen (1977) and Shock (1974).

Cellular Theories
Of Aging

In the early part of this century, it was widely believed that if some cells were not immortal, at the very least they could grow and multiply for an extended time. Child (1915) "showed" that senescence in planarians (small flatworms which move by means of cilia) is reversible, while Carrel (1912) "demonstrated" that tissue cells taken from adult animals could be propagated indefinitely *in vitro* (in a test tube or other artificial environment). In the same vein, Bidder (1925, 1932) "identified" a number of instances in fish where the lifespan was not believed to be fixed—that is, general vigor appeared to persist indefinitely.

Recent experiments, particularly those observing cell growth and development in tissue culture, suggest that this earlier research was inaccurate. Leonard Hayflick has shown that normal human fibroblasts (embryonic cells that give rise to connective tissue) cultured *in vitro* undergo a limited number of divisions and then die. Hayflick and Moorehead (1961) observed that such cells undergo fifty divisions *in vitro* before losing the ability to replicate themselves. In 1965, Hayflick reported that fibroblasts isolated from human adult tissue undergo only about 20 divisions *in vitro*. One the basis of these and other studies he argued that (1) the limited replicative capacity of cultured normal human cells is an expression of programmed genetic events and (2) the limit on normal cell division *in vitro* is a function of the age of the donor. Thus it is now generally believed that there is an inverse relationship between the age of a human donor and the *in vitro* cell division capacity of fibroblasts derived from the skin, lungs and liver (Hayflick, 1977).

While it appears that normal cells have a finite lifetime, this is not the case for "abnormal cells." Such cells, which are structurally and/or genetically distinguishable from normal cells, are capable of unlimited division. Cancer cells, for example, are able to divide indefinitely in tissue culture. A famous line of human cancer cells named Hela (after Henrietta Lacks, the woman from whom they were taken before her death in 1951) is still being cultured for use in standardized cancer cell studies (Gold, 1981). Whatever causes noncancerous cells to gradually lose the ability to divide appears to be lacking in cancer cells. The study of cancer may yet reveal what limits the ability of normal cells to divide indefinitely.

Hayflick is not alone in arguing that aging is genetically programmed into cells. Bernard Strehler of the University of Southern California has hypothesized that programmed loss of genetic material could cause aging. As Strehler (1973) points out, most cells contain hundreds of repetitions of the same DNA (the molecule of heredity in nearly all organisms) for the known genes they contain. This simply means that the cell does not have to rely upon a single copy of its genetic blueprint for any one trait. In experiments done on beagles, Strehler found that as cells age, a considerable number of these repetitions are lost (Johnson, Crisp and Strehler, 1972). This is especially true for brain, heart and skeletal muscle cells. How the loss occurs is not specifically known, though there is some speculation that it results from age-related changes in cell metabolism. Strehler suspects that cells may be programmed, at a fixed point in life, to start manufacturing a substance that inhibits protein synthesis.

Vincent Cristafalo of the Wistar Institute in Philadelphia has studied the relationship between aging and cell metabolism in human fibroblasts. Of particular interest to him are lysosomes, which are sac-like structures in the cell cytoplasm. They contain digestive enzymes that implement the breakdown of fats, proteins and nucleic acids. It is thought that lysosomes serve to isolate these digestive enzymes from the cell cytoplasm, thereby keeping the cell from ingesting itself. Cristafalo has found that the number of lysosomes in the cell cytoplasm increases as cells age. When a lysosome membrane is ruptured, the cell undergoes chemical breakdown; aging could be a result of the perforation of lysosome membranes. Cristafalo (1975) added hydrocortisone, a drug thought to increase the stability of lysosome membranes, to cultures of human fibroblast cells. He found that the presence of this drug increased the life span of the cells by 30 to 40 percent. However, since hydrocortisone stimulates protein synthesis in cells, it is possible that it is the relationship between these two which is responsible for the increased longevity of the cells in Christafalo's experiments, not the relationship between hydrocortisone and the stability of lysosome membranes.

Another school of thought claims that senescence is largely a result of the accumulation of accidental changes that occur in cells over a period of time. F. Marott Sinex (1977) of the Boston University School of Medicine believes that random mutations may produce aging by causing damage to DNA molecules. Although the cell has DNA repair mechanisms, it is likely that either some mutational changes are too subtle for the repair process to detect or that mutations occur too rapidly for them all to be repaired. Apparently, it is theorized, as the mutations accumulate in the body's cells, the cells begin to lose their ability to function, including perhaps even a loss of the ability to divide. This mutation theory is not incompatible with the theory of genetic programming. It is certainly plausible that a shutoff of the DNA repair mechanism is a programmed genetic event.

While these theories are concerned with aging at the cellular level, it is a large leap from cell biology to a consideration of aging in the total organism. There are several physiological theories which attempt to relate aging to the performance of the total organism.

Physiological Theories
Of Aging

One physiological theory of aging involves the autoimmune mechanism. This theory postulates that because of "copying errors" in repeated cell divisions, protein enzymes produced by newer cells may not be recognized by the body.

As a result, the body's immunological system would be brought into play, forcing the body to work against itself. Rheumatoid arthritis, a chronic, inflammatory disease that can lead to bone dislocation, joint fusion, and great pain and discomfort, is popularly believed to be a consequence of autoimmunity. Two different explanations are generally offered to explain autoimmune reactions. One is that the body somehow comes to regard its own tissue as a foreign substance and responds accordingly—antibodies are produced that work against the body in some way. A second explanation posits that rheumatoid arthritis is a result of a preexisting foreign substance (antigen) or infectious microorganism and its specific antibody response. This second explanation maintains that the antigen-antibody complex settles in highly vascular tissue (this is tissue with a high concentration of vessels for carrying blood or lymph such as membranes between joints) and that subsequently the complex somehow acts as an antigen itself and perpetuates an inflammatory response (Kart, Metress and Metress, 1978). The autoimmune phenomenon appears to increase with age (Sigel and Good, 1972), though it is not clear whether this results from the increased "copying errors" that come with age or from the aging of the immunological system itself.

Another theory with a long history is the "wear and tear" theory of aging. In effect, this theory posits an inverse relationship between "rate of living" and length of life—that is, those who live too hard and fast cannot expect to live very long. In the early part of this century, Rubner (described in Comfort, 1979) carried out calorimetric experiments to determine the energy requirements necessary for the maintenance of body metabolism. He suggested that senescence might reflect the expenditure of fixed amounts of energy used to complete particular chemical reactions. An important question then arises: Can an individual live a life which causes a speedup or slowdown in the expenditure of such energy?

Many theorists employing the wear and tear model use machine analogies to demonstrate the theory's underlying assumptions that an organism wears out with use. However, these analogies often fail to take into account two important characteristics of living organisms: (1) living organisms have mechanisms for self-repair not available to machines; and (2) functions in a living organism may actually become more efficient with use.

Hans Selye's work on stress has been used by some to support the wear and tear theory. Based on experiments with animals, Selye (1966) has identified three stages of response to continued stress. Each stage of response parallels a phase of aging. Stage one is characterized by an alarm reaction in which the body's adaptive forces are being activated but are not yet fully operational. This stage is reminiscent of childhood, a period during which adaptability to stress is growing, but in which adaptability is still limited. Stage two is the stage of resistance—mobilization of the defensive reactions to stress is completed. This parallels adulthood, during which the body has acquired resistance to most stress agents likely to affect it. Stage three, the stage of exhaustion, eventually results in a breakdown of resistance and eventual death. This last stage parallels the process of senescence in human beings.

Though it makes intuitive sense that an old animal is less able to withstand the same stress that can be tolerated by a young animal, there is little empirical evidence that accumulated stress is the cause of aging. Selye's work has been and continues to be important in showing the relationship between stress and disease. However it has not yet been helpful in attempts to specify the mechanisms of aging.

Collagen, a protein fiber, has also been implicated in age-related changes in physiological functions. Collagen constitutes about 30 percent of the body's protein and is distributed in and around the walls of blood vessels and in connective tissue. With age, collagen shows a reduction in its elastic properties. According to the collagen theory of aging, alteration in this protein fiber plays an important role in impairing functional capacities. For example, the reduced efficiency of cardiac muscle may be the result of increasing stiffness. Connective tissue changes in small blood vessels may lead to the development of hypertension. Even cell permeability may be affected, making it more difficult for cells to acquire nutrients and expel wastes.

Nathan Shock (1974), a noted gerontologist, has recently suggested that there is sufficient evidence for us to entertain the possibility that aging results from some breakdown or impairment in the performance of endocrine and/or neural control mechanisms. Studies carried out by the National Institute of Health's Gerontology Research Center show that age-related declines in humans are greater for functions which are complex and require the coordinated activity of whole organ systems. Measurements of functions related to a single physiological system, like nerve conduction velocity, show considerably less age decrement than do functions such as maximum breathing capacity, which involve coordination between systems (in this case between the nervous and muscular systems).

The relationship between age and task performance efficiency also shows an age-related decline that is most likely associated with task complexity. For example, simple motor performance, as demonstrated by the time it takes an individual to push a button in response to a signal of light, increases only modestly across the human life span. Complex motor performance, on the other hand, does show significant decrement with age. Complex motor performance can involve having an individual select one of several possible responses after the presentation of a complex stimulus. While simple motor performance involves the transmission of nerve impulses over short distances and through relatively few synapses, complex motor performance requires transmission through many synapses and is influenced by other factors in the central nervous system. Interestingly, though, the aged often show significantly improved motor performance with practice (Botwinick, 1973).

PROLONGEVITY

A number of the theories of biological aging discussed above raise issues about the role of adequate nutrition in achieving long life. For example. theories at both the cellular level (Cristafalo) and the physiological level (autoimmune theory) recognize the possible link between protein synthesis and the aging process. Diet plays a role in protein synthesis by supplying the nutrients necessary for normal enzyme activity and production. Not only may diet affect cellular and physiological processes but, as we have indicated, nutrition plays a part in the course of degenerative diseases that often accompany aging. More will be said about this in Chapter 6. Much more research is needed on the impact of proper nutrition and diet supplementation on the aging process.

Whether or not diet can directly affect longevity is still subject to considerable debate. Most research in this area has been carried out on various species of animals. In general, underfeeding seems to increase longevity, although the biological mechanisms responsible for this are unknown. One exception to this involves underfeeding during the perinatal period. Roeder (1973) effected perinatal undernutrition in rats and observed biochemical changes that she interpreted as indications of accelerated aging.

Underfed animals showing increased longevity also show reduced incidence and severity, and a delay in the age of onset, of various diseases. Berg and Simms (1962) reduced the dietary intake of rats by 46 percent. This was accompanied by a 25 percent increase in life span and a delay in the age at which 40 percent of the animals had chronic glomerulonephritis (inflammation of the filtering structures in the kidney that help form urine). Again, the biological mechanisms that bring about these results remain unknown.

Some information presented in this chapter may lead readers to believe that because the length of human life has been increased, it will continue to increase almost automatically as a by-product of technological and social changes. Whether or not this is really so is unclear and points up the necessity of distinguishing between the concepts "life expectancy" and "life span." While life expectancy refers to the average length of life of persons, life span refers to the longevity of long-lived persons. Life span is the extreme limit of human longevity, the age beyond which no one can expect to live (Gruman, 1977:7). Gerontologists estimate the life span to be about 110 years; some have argued that it has not increased notably in the course of history (Dublin, 1957; Sacher and Havighurst, n.d.).

Is the human life span an absolute standard? Or can (should) we expect a significant extension of the length of life? Some have always shared the view that human life should be lengthened indefinitely. These are proponents of *prolongevity*, which is defined as the significant extension of the length of life by human action (Gruman, 1977:6). Others believe that new treatments and technology as well as improved health habits may continue to increase life expectancy but that human life span is unlikely to increase.

Prolongevitists often point to the "long-lived" peoples in mountain regions of Ecuador (the Andean village of Vilacabamba), Pakistan (the Hunza people of Kashmir), and the Soviet Union (the Abkhasians in the Russian Caucasus) as examples of populations that have already extended the human life span (Leaf, 1973). However, many find reports on the world's long-lived peoples to be self-serving, and their suspicions are heightened by the writings of experts such as the Russan gerontologist Medvedev (1974), who offers an explanation of why many in the Caucasus claim superlongevity:

The famous man from Yakutia, who was found during the 1959 census to be 130 years old, received especially great publicity because he lived in the place with the most terrible climate. (This place is sometimes called the Pole of Cold, because the winter temperature here is about − 50 C to − 60 C.) When publicity about him became all-national and a large article with a picture of this outstanding man was published in the central government newspaper, *Isvestia*, the puzzle was quickly solved. A letter was received from a group of Ukrainian villagers who recognized this centenarian as a fellow villager who deserted from the army during the First World War and forged documents or used his father's (most usual method of falsification) to escape remobilization. It was found that this man was really only 78 years old.

Still, there is considerable interest—even mass interest—in increasing human longevity. A good part of this interest originates in the antediluvian theme found in tradition and folklore that people lived much longer in the distant past. Noah, after all, supposedly lived to be 950 years old.

What are the prospects for continued reduction in death rates and life extension? As we have already shown (Table 1.3), death rates have declined and are likely to continue to do so. However, some research suggests that there is little room for improvement, unless some significant breakthrough eliminates cardiovascular diseases. In any case, small improvements would seem to be attainable. According to Siegel (1975), if the lowest death rates for females in the countries of Europe are combined into a single table, the values for life expectancy at birth and at age sixty-five exceed those same values for the U.S. by 4.3 and 1.4 years respectively. Table 1.6 shows average life expectancy at birth, according to sex, for selected countries in the years 1972 and 1977. Using the data for 1977, it is clear that Canada, Denmark, France, Netherlands, Sweden, Switzerland and Japan have life expectancies at birth for both males and females that exceed those of the United States.

Most elderly people die as a result of some long-standing chronic condition, which is sometimes related to personal habits (for example, smoking, drinking, poor eating habits) or environmental conditions (for example, harsh work environments, air pollution) that go back many years. Attempts to prevent illness and death from these conditions must begin before old age. But what if we could prevent deaths from these conditions? Table 1.7 gives a partial answer to this question. The elimination of all deaths in the United States caused by accidents, influenza and pneumonia, infective and parasitic diseases, diabetes mellitus, and tuberculosis would increase life expectancy at birth by 2.2 years and at age sixty-five by 0.7 years. Even the elimination of cancer as a cause of death would result in only a 2.3 year gain in life expectancy at birth and about half that at age sixty-five. This is because cancer affects individuals in all age groups. If the major cardiovascular-renal diseases were eliminated, there would be a 10.9 year gain in life expectancy at birth, and even a 10.0 year gain in life expectancy at age sixty-five. These diseases are not likely to be eliminated in the near future, although death rates as a result of them may be reduced.

Where there is substantial room for improvement in death rates and life expectancies in the United States is among men and nonwhites. As has already been pointed out in this chapter (table 1.2), the death rate for men sixty-five years of age and older was 46 percent higher than that of elderly women in 1976. In 1977, among those aged sixty-five to sixty-nine, black males had a death rate from all causes that was 15 percent higher than that of white males. Black females had a death rate 37 percent higher than their white counterparts.

TABLE 1.6.   Life expectancy at birth, according to sex: Selected countries, 1972 and 1977. (Data are based on reporting by countries.)

	MALE			FEMALE		
COUNTRY	1972[1]	1977[2]	AVERAGE ANNUAL CHANGE IN YEARS	1972[1]	1977[2]	AVERAGE ANNUAL CHANGE IN YEARS
	Life expectancy in years			Life expectancy in years		
Canada............	69.3	69.8	0.2	76.7	77.3	0.2
United States.......	67.4	69.3	0.4	75.1	77.1	0.4
Austria	66.9	68.5	0.3	74.1	75.5	0.3
Denmark...........	70.8	71.9	0.2	76.3	78.0	0.3
England and Wales ..	69.0	70.2	0.2	75.3	76.3	0.2
France	69.1	69.9	0.2	77.1	77.9	0.2
German Democratic Republic.........	68.9	68.9	–	74.2	74.5	0.1
German Federal Republic.........	67.6	69.2	0.3	74.2	76.0	0.4
Ireland	68.5	69.0	0.2	73.4	74.3	0.3
Italy...............	68.9	69.9	0.3	75.2	76.1	0.3
Netherlands........	70.9	72.2	0.3	76.9	78.8	0.4
Sweden...........	72.1	72.8	0.1	77.7	79.2	0.3
Switzerland	70.7	72.1	0.3	77.0	79.0	0.4
Israel[3]	70.7	71.4	0.1	73.2	74.8	0.3
Japan.............	70.8	72.9	0.4	76.3	78.2	0.4
Australia...........	67.4	70.0	0.4	74.2	77.0	0.4
New Zealand	68.6	68.9	0.1	74.6	75.4	0.2

[1]Data for the German Democratic Republic refer to the average for the period 1969-70; data for Australia refer to 1970; data for New Zealand refer to the average for the period 1970-72.

[2]Data for Canada, Ireland, Italy and New Zealand refer to 1975; data for the German Democratic Republic and France refer to 1976.

[3]Jewish population only for 1972.

Source: U.S. Department of Health and Human Services, Health, United States, 1980. DHHS Publication No. (PHS) 81-1232, Table 13, p. 136, Washington, D.C., U.S. Government Printing Office, December, 1980.

TABLE 1.7.   Gain in expectation of life at birth and at age 65 due to elimination of various causes of death: United States, 1959-1961.

VARIOUS CAUSES OF DEATH	AT BIRTH	TOTAL AT AGE 65
Major cardiovascular-renal diseases	10.9	10.0
Diseases of the heart	5.9	4.9
Stroke	1.3	1.2
Malignant neoplasms (cancers)	2.3	1.2
All accidents excluding motor vehicles	0.6	0.1
Motor vehicle accidents	0.6	0.1
Influenza and pneumonia	0.5	0.2
Infective and parasitic diseases	0.2	0.1
Diabetes mellitus	0.2	0.2
Tuberculosis	0.1	–

Source: Siegel, 1975, Table 16.

Much more public discussion of biogerontological research on prolongevity is needed. Improving death rates and life expectancies in the U.S. along the lines suggested above would still not achieve an extension of the life span. Should people live to be 120 or 130 years of age? When thinking about your answer, assume first that this would involve more than a simple increase in time at the end of life. Imagine that researchers could alter the rate of aging in such a way as to give extra years to the healthy and productive stages of life. Under these conditions, extra years might be difficult to turn down. But, what if a longer life meant a longer "old age?" Many of you, while thinking of answers to the question of whether we should extend the human life span, will think about pollution, overpopulation, dwindling energy resources, retirement policies, social security benefits and the like. The list is a long one.

SUMMARY

Holding off death, prolonging life, has been a prominent theme in the past as well as in contemporary times. This is reflected in the antediluvian, hyperborean, and fountain themes, each of which may be used to suggest a positive relationship between nutrition and aging or longevity.

Students of the as yet "unfinished" sciences of nutrition and gerontology have identified at least three points where the two sciences intersect. These intersections set the parameters of the emerging field of geriatric nutrition. They include the role of nutrition in biological aging, the relationship between nutrition and disease, and the relationship between the social context of aging and nutrition.

A number of variables influence the time in life when we show the kind of vulnerability to aging processes that result in death. These include not only differences in biological potential but also social and environmental factors. Men have higher death rates than women in every age category, and blacks (up to eighty years of age) have higher death rates than whites. However, age-adjusted death rates in the total population in 1977 dropped to about one-third of what they were in 1900.

Biogerontologists have attempted to answer the question, "Why do we become old?" at both the cellular and physiological levels. More research on this question is needed. Attempts must be made to test the relative merits of the genetic programming and mutation theory, as well as the collagen and stress theory. Also, perhaps the expectation that one explanation exists for the phenomenon of biological aging should be abandoned. Aging is a complex phenomenon and it may well be that different explanations are required for different aspects of the aging process.

Finally, what if we solve the riddle of biological aging? Should we welcome prolongevity? And have we thought sufficiently about its potential impact on individuals as well as on society as a whole?

STUDY QUESTIONS

1. Describe the antediluvian, hyperborean, and fountain themes of aging. How are these themes reflected in present day society?
2. Identify three intersections where the study of aging and the study of nutrition meet.
3. What is the impact of race on mortality rates in America today? What role do socioeconomic factors play in this relationship? Of what import is all of this to understanding the relationship between nutrition and aging?
4. Define the term *senescence.* How does senescence differ from other biological processes?
5. Explain the relationship between sex and mortality. (Remember to distinguish between biological and socioenvironmental explanations.)
6. Identify two currently popular cellular theories of aging. How do these theories differ from those posited in the early part of the twentieth century?
7. Describe and contrast the autoimmune, collagen, and wear-and-tear theories of aging.
8. Distinguish between the concepts of "life span" and "life expectancy."
9. Define *prolongevity.* Discuss some possible consequences (for the individual *and* society) of a significant extension of the human life span.

BIBLIOGRAPHY

American Cancer Society, *Cancer Facts and Figures.* New York, American Cancer Society, 1978.

BAKER, J. and ALLEN, G., *The Study of Biology* (Third Edition). Menlo Park, Calif., Addison-Wesley, 1977.

BENET, S., "Why They Live to be 100, or Even Older in Abkhasia," *The New York Times Magazine*, December 26, 1971.

————, *Abkhasians: The Long-Lived People of the Caucasus*. New York, Holt, Rinehart & Winston, Inc., 1974.

BERG, B. and SIMMS, H.S., "Relation of Nutrition to Longevity and Onset of Disease in Rats," in *Biological Aspects of Aging*, ed. by N. Shock. New York, Columbia University Press, 1962.

BIDDER, G. P., "The Mortality of Plaice," *Nature*, 115 (1925), 495.

————, "Senescence," *British Medical Journal*, 115 (1932), 5831.

BOGUE, D. J., *Principles of Demography*. New York, John Wiley, 1969.

BOTWINICK, J., *Aging and Behavior: A Comprehensive Integration of Research Findings*. New York, Springer-Verlag, 1973.

CAMUS, A., *The Myth of Sisyphus and Other Essays*. New York, Knopf, 1955.

CARREL, A., "On the Permanent Life of Tissues," *Journal of Experimental Medicine*, 15, (1912), 516.

CHILD, C. M., *Senescence and Rejuvenescence*. Chicago, University of Chicago Press, 1915.

COMFORT, A., *The Biology of Senescence* (Third Edition). New York, Elsevier, 1979.

CRISTAFALO, V., "Hydrocortisone as a Modulator of Cell Division and Population Life Span," in *Explorations in Aging*, ed. by V. Cristafalo, J. Roberts, and R. Adelman. New York, Plenum, 1975.

DORN, H., "Mortality," in *The Study of Population*, ed. by P. Hauser and O. Duncan. Chicago, University of Chicago Press, 1959.

DUBLIN, L. I., "Outlook for Longevity in the United States," *Newsletter, Gerontology Society*, 4, no. 2 (1957), 3.

GOLD, M., "The Cells That Would Not Die," *Science 81*, 2, no. 3 (April 1981), 28–35.

GONNELLA, J. S., LOUIS, D. Z., and McCORD, J. J., "The Staging Concept: An Approach to the Assessment of Outcome of Ambulatory Care," *Medical Care*, 14 (1976), 13–21.

GRUMAN, G., *A History of Ideas About the Prolongation of Life*. Philadelphia, Pa., American Philosophical Society, 1966.

————, *A History of Ideas About the Prolongation of Life*. New York, Arno, 1977.

HAYFLICK, L., "The Limited *in vitro* Lifetime of Human Diploid Cell Strains," *Experimental Cell Research*, 37 (1965), 614–636.

————, "The Cellular Basis for Biological Aging," in *Handbook of the Biology of Aging*, ed. by C. Finch and L. Hayflick. New York, Van Nostrand Reinhold, 1977.

———— and Moorehead, P.S., "The Serial Cultivation of Human Diploid Cell Strains," *Experimental Cell Research*, 25 (1961), 585–621.

JOHNSON, R., CRISP, C., and STREHLER, B., "Selective Loss of Ribosomal RNA Genes During the Aging of Post-Mitotic Tissues," *Mechanisms of Aging and Development*, 1 (1972).

KART, C., METRESS, E., and METRESS, J., *Aging and Health*. Menlo Park, California, Addison-Wesley, 1978.

KITAGAWA, E. and HAUSER, P. M., *Differential Mortality in the United States: A Study in Scientific Epidemiology*. Cambridge, Mass., Harvard University Press, 1973.

KYNCHARYANTS, V., "Will the Human Life-Span Reach One Hundred?" *Gerontologist*, 14 (1974), 377–380.

LEAF, A., "Getting Old," *Scientific American*, 229, no. 3 (1973), 44–52.

MADIGAN, F., "Are Sex Mortality Differentials Biologically Caused?" *Milbank Memorial Fund Quarterly*, 35, no. 2 (1957), 202–223.

MAYER, J., *Health*. New York, D. Van Nostrand Co., 1974.

MEDVEDEV, Z. A., "Caucasus and Altay Longevity: A Biological or Social Problem?" *Gerontologist*, 14 (1974), 381–387.

_____, "Aging and Longevity: New Approaches and New Perspectives," *Gerontologist*, 15 (1975), 196–201.

PETERSEN, W., *Population* (Third Edition). New York, Macmillan, 1975.

ROEDER, L., "Effect of the Level of Nutrition on Rates of Cell Proliferation and of RNA and Protein Synthesis in the Rat," *Nutrition Reports International*, 7 (1973), 271–288.

SACHER, G. A. and HAVIGHURST, R. J., "Prospects of Lengthening Life and Vigor," Unpublished Manuscript, n.d.

SELYE, H., *The Stress of Life* (Second Edition). New York, McGraw-Hill, 1966.

SHOCK, N., "Physiological Theories of Aging," in *Theoretical Aspects of Aging*, ed. by M. Rockstein. New York, Academic Press, 1974.

SIEGEL, J. S., "Some Demographic Aspects of Aging in the United States," in *Epidemiology of Aging*, ed. by A. Ostfeld and D. Gibson. Bethesda, Md., National Institute of Health, 1975.

_____, *Prospective Trends in the Size and Structure of the Elderly Population, Impact of Mortality Trends, and Some Implications*. Current Population Reports, Special Studies Series P-23, No. 78. Washington, D.C., U.S. Department of Commerce, Bureau of the Census, 1979.

SIGEL, M. and GOOD, R., *Tolerance, Autoimmunity and Aging*. Springfield, Ill., Charles C Thomas, 1972.

SINEX, F. M., "The Molecular Genetics of Aging," in *Handbook of the Biology of Aging*, ed. by C. Finch and L. Hayflick. New York, Van Nostrand Reinhold, 1977.

STREHLER, B., *Time, Cells and Aging*. New York, Academic Press, 1962.

_____, "A New Age for Aging," *Natural History*, February, 1973.

United States Office of Health Resources Opportunity, *Health Status of Minorities and Low-Income Groups*. DHEW Pub. No. (HRA) 79–627. Health Resources Administration, Washington, D.C., U.S. Government Printing Office, 1979.

CHAPTER TWO
THE GRAYING
OF AMERICA

In addition to biological factors, social and economic considerations such as marital status, income, health, and housing arrangements may directly or indirectly affect an elderly person's health and nutritional status. Some of these relationships are quite complicated. For instance, an older person who has low income may be unable to maintain an adequate dietary regimen, but even someone with a high income, in the presence of "aloneness," may have no added protection from malnourishment. Pulitzer prize winner Robert Butler (1975:145) reports the following case:

> A 95-year-old retired corporation executive lived in an exclusive apartment complex. He had outlived friends and relatives. He had an income over $900 a month and $300,000 in assets, yet he was starving to death. His memory had become hazy and he forgot his mealtimes. No one realized he was subsisting on a few sweets and tea.

Specific relationships between factors such as income and the nutritional status of elderly people will be discussed in Chapter 5. In the present chapter, some demographic characteristics of the aged population are described. In doing so, we reveal the important statistical dimensions of the aged population and make projections within limits about its future. An important implication of this statistical presentation is that nutrition problems among the aged can result from the particular social and economic characteristics that they share as a group. After all, people who are old today share a common history. They have experienced historical events similarly—that is, at about the same age. In addition, their behaviors and attitudes (even those related to food and nutrition) have been shaped by these experiences, which serve to distinguish them from those who will be old twenty or thirty years from now.

Before beginning, several caveats are in order. First, in the present discussion, the age range of 65 and over is used as the basis for identifying and describing the elderly population. Much of the available data in the United States defines the elderly as those 65 years of age and over, and though this is an imprecise identifier of the older population, we follow it in this chapter. Second, while as a group the elderly population is markedly different in its socioeconomic characteristics from that group which composes the younger population, it is important to remember that despite a common history, the elderly are not a homogeneous group. They are as diverse a population as are those in younger age groups. If we were to compare younger old people (those aged 65 to 74, for example) with the *"old-old"* (those 75 years and older), we would find sharp differences with respect to work status, income, marital status, and living arrangements.

The final caveat, related to the above point, is the fact that summary statistical measures are often used in describing the characteristics of a population. It is important to recognize that these measures represent statistical generalizations that can hide the wide variation that exists within a population. For example, while it may be reported that the median annual income for families headed by an older person was $10,140 in 1978, you should remember that the yearly income of Ronald Reagan's family was far in excess of this amount.

NUMBER AND PROPORTION
OF THE ELDERLY

The elderly population of the United States has grown consistently during this century. In 1900, there were approximately 3 million men and women aged 65 and over; by 1980, this population had increased to almost 25 million (see Table 2.1). This more than eightfold gain represents a rate of increase substantially greater than the rate of increase for the total population, which less than tripled from 76 to 221 million in the same period. Between now and the end of the century, the elderly population is expected to continue to grow albeit at a slower rate. However, the aged are still expected to increase in number to about 32 million in the year 2000 and to about 45 million in 2020 (more than double the 1970 elderly population).

As Table 2.1 indicates, the rate of increase in the elderly population from the preceding decade is expected to peak in the 1970–1980 decade and decline until the 2010–2020 decade. Note, for example, that between 1990 and 2000

TABLE 2.1. Total aged population and percent of the total population which is aged: 1960–2020[1]

YEAR	1960	1970	1980	1990	2000	2010	2020
Elderly Pop. (65 +) (000)	16,675	20,087	24,927	29,824	31,822	34,837	45,102
Percent of Total Population 65 +	9.3	9.9	11.2	12.2	12.2	12.7	15.5
Increase in Preceding Decade (Percent)	—	20.5	24.1	19.6	6.7	9.5	29.5

[1]1960–1970 are estimates; 1980–2020 are based on Series II Census Bureau Projections. These projections are based on three assumptions: (1) an average of 2.1 children born to a woman in her lifetime; (2) a moderate decline in mortality; and (3) net immigration of 400,000 per year.

Source: Siegel, J. *Prospective Trends in the Size and Structure of the Elderly Population, Impact of Mortality Trends, and Some Implications* (CPR Special Studies Series P–23, No. 78). Bureau of the Census, 1979.

the projected population increase for the elderly is only about two million, or a 6.7 percent decennial increase. This compares with the 4.8 million or 24.1 percent decennial increase projected between 1970 and 1980. Also, between 1990 and 2000 we can observe the aged as constituting a stable proportion of the total population—12.2 percent.

This slowed rate of increase in the ratio of the elderly to the total population is a reflection of the low birth rates during the economic depression through World War II. For example, those born in 1929 will reach age 65 during the last decade of this century. When the "postwar" babies—those born just after 1945—reach age 65, shortly after 2010, the elderly population will again increase. Table 2.1 shows the projected increase in the elderly population between 2010 and 2020 to be 29.5 percent. This growth rate will probably fall again by about 2030. This is because of the current continuing decline in birth rates that began in the 1960s.

Just how accurate are these estimations of the size of the future older population? United States Census Bureau projections of the population sixty-five years of age and over for 1975 were published at various dates from August 1953 until December 1972 and varied from 20.7 million to 22.2 million. The current estimate is 22.4 million, 7.9 percent above the low estimate and 1.1 percent above the high estimate. As Siegel (1979) points out, the percent deviation from the current estimate declined as the publication date approached 1975. This is what might be expected. The first projections were made about a future that was twenty-two years away; in December of 1972, this future was only three years ahead.

This phenomenon has already appeared in projections for the year 2000. Until 1975, estimates for the older population of 2000 were in the 28–29 million range. In 1975, the Census Bureau increased the estimate to about 30.5 million. The latest projection is four percent greater, or 31.8 million people aged sixty-five and over in the year 2000. According to Siegel, these newly revised estimates reflect lower than anticipated mortality rates in the 1972-76 period and the subsequent use of more favorable mortality rates in making future estimates.

What proportion of the total population older people will comprise in the future will be determined in great part by fertility (birth rate) levels. It is likely that severely depressed fertility rates will increase the proportion of the older population to about 17 percent by the year 2020; a new "baby boom" would put it somewhere between 12 and 13 percent in 2020. A projection somewhere in between (and accepted by many) would be about 15 percent in 2020.

THE DEPENDENCY RATIO

The growth of the elderly population has led gerontologists to look at the demographic relationship between this group and the rest of the population. To some, this relationship suggests the size of the burden a society will feel in supporting its elderly members. One crude measure used to summarize this demographic relationship is known as the *dependency ratio*. Arithmetically, the ratio represents the number or proportion of individuals in the dependent segment of the population divided by the number or proportion of individuals in the supportive or working population. While the dependent population has two components, the young *and* the old, gerontologists are especially concerned with the *old-age dependency ratio*. Definitions of "old" and "working" are "65 and over" and "18 to 64" years of age respectively. Thus the old-age dependency ratio is, in simple demographic terms, $65+/18-64$. This does not mean that every person aged 65 and over is dependent or that every person in the 18 to 64 range is working. These basic census categories are only used to depict the numerical relationship between these two segments of a society's population.

Table 2.2 shows old-age dependency ratios for the United States from 1930 to 2020. Though the ratio has increased in this century, it is expected to change very little between 1975 and 2010. Note that in the second decade of the next century the ratio rises again. The *baby-boom* children of the 1940s and 1950s will have reached retirement age, thus increasing the numerator, and a lowered birth rate, such as we have now, means a relatively smaller work force population (18–64), reducing the denominator (Cutler and Harootyan, 1975). The projected old-age dependency ratio of .26 in 2020 indicates that every individual 65 years of age or over will hypothetically be supported by four working persons between the ages of 18 and 64; in 1930, this ratio was about one to ten.

Some demographers distinguish between a "societal" old-age dependency ratio (just discussed) and a "familial" old-age dependency ratio. The familial old-age dependency ratio can be used to crudely illustrate the shifts in the ratio of elderly parents to the children who would support them. This ratio is also defined in simple demographic terms using the formula: population 65–79/population 45–49. This does not mean that all persons aged 65–79 need support (or even have children) or that every person in the 45–49 age range is willing or able to provide. However, we use these census age categories to depict the ratio of the number of elderly persons to the number of younger persons of the next generation.

Table 2.2 also shows familial old-age dependency ratios for the United States from 1930 to 2020. The ratios increased from 1930 on and reached a peak in 1980. In 1930, there were 82 persons 65–79 years of age for every 100 persons aged 45–49. This figure was 156 in 1976 and was expected to reach 180 by 1980. A higher figure of 216 is projected for 2020.

Changes in the familial old-age dependency ratio result mainly from past trends in fertility. For example, the high ratio expected in 1980 reflects the combination of high fertility (and migration) in the early part of this century (population 65–79) and reduced birth rates during the 1930s (population 45–49). The high ratio expected in the year 2020 results from high fertility

TABLE 2.2.   Old-age dependency ratios for the United States, 1930–2020.

YEAR	OLD-AGE DEPENDENCY RATIOS[1]	FAMILIAL-OLD AGE DEPENDENCY RATIOS[2]
1930	.09	.82
1940	.11	.95
1950	.13	1.16
1960	.17	1.29
1970	.17	1.35
1975	.18	
Projections		
1980	.18	1.80
1990	.20	1.68
2000	.20	1.25
2010	.20	1.27
2020	.26	2.16

[1]Old-Age Dependency Ratio = 65+/18–64
[2]Familial-Old Age Dependency Ratio = pop. 65–79/pop. 45–49

Sources: U.S. Bureau fo the Census, Demographic Aspects of Aging and the Older Population in the United States (Series P-23, No. 59), and Projections of the Population of the United States: 1977–2050 (Series P-25, No. 704).

rates during the post–World War II baby-boom years and lower birth rates in the early 1970s.

How will these changes in the familial old-age dependency ratio affect family life in the future for aged persons? Many of the elderly receive considerable social and economic support from their children and other relatives. However, pessimists suggest that there may be demographic limits on such support. Treas (1977) points out that the limitations of the family support system are already spawning a service industry and a professional corps to provide regular meals, housekeeping services, and institutionalized care. This trend is expected to continue, but at a slowed pace until about 2010. People who are old today formed their families during the 1930s and had an average of three children. People who will be old in the latter part of this century (up to about 2000) will have more children and relatives due to the baby boom and the more recent lower mortality rates. Those who become old in the twenty-first century will have had two or less children on the average and may be unable to look to the family for support. In addition, unless the future aged are better able to support themselves than are current cohorts of the elderly, we may expect the role of government to expand in providing health and other support services to the aged.

Another view is more optimistic. Many persons who are old today have aged parents who are still living. Increased longevity would make this phenomenon more pronounced in the future. The four-or-five generation family may be the norm in the next century. Children may come to know great-grandparents and even great-great grandparents (Neugarten, 1975). This could make possible more intergenerational households and, thus, more family support.

AGE AND SEX COMPOSITION

While America's older population has grown in size and proportion to the total population during this century, its average age has increased as well. The proportion of the aged who are 65–69 years of age (some of the "young old" has been and will continue to get smaller; the proportion 75 and over has been getting larger, and this trend is expected to continue. In 1900, the proportion of those 65 years of age and over who were 75 or over was 20 percent. By the year 2000, this figure will be about 43 percent.

Typically, elderly women outnumber elderly men. This is because at virtually all ages the number of male deaths exceeds the number of female deaths. The disparity between the number of elderly men and women has been growing for several decades. In 1960, the number of males for every 100 females, or the *sex ratio*, was 82.6 in the over-65 population. By 1979 this ratio had declined to 68.4. The sex ratio of the older population is projected to decline further to 66.6 by 2000.

NATIVITY AND RACE

Blacks make up the largest racial minority among older people. A much smaller proportion of the black population is 65 and over than is the case for the white population. In 1978, the black elderly made up about 7.5 percent of the total black population. The "youthfulness" of the black population is a consequence of their higher fertility rate. The lower life expectancy of blacks relative to whites (discussed in Chapter 1) contributes only moderately to the youthfulness of this population.

In 1976, Spanish Americans constituted about 5.3 percent of the U.S. population amounting to over 11 million people. The elderly among them account for about 4 percent of their total number. By and large, the same reasons mentioned for the youthfulness of the black population apply to this group. A higher fertility rate and reduced life expectancy both contribute to the reduced size of the elderly Hispanic population. In addition, immigration of the young and some repatriation of the middle-aged contribute to the youthfulness of this ethnic group.

The sex ratio among aged blacks is higher than that for aged whites. This is generally thought to reflect a narrower gap between nonwhite male and female mortality rates than is the case for whites. For example, in 1979, there were 3.2 more men per 100 women among blacks 65 years of age and over than there were for whites.

HEALTH STATUS

While human organs gradually diminish in function over time, such loss does not occur at the same rate in every individual. This gradual diminishing of function by itself is not a real threat to the health status of most older people. Diseases represent the chief barriers to extended health and longevity. When the potential for disease is superimposed on the normal changes associated with biological aging, maintaining health becomes especially problematic for older people.

In the Unites States today, chronic conditions represent the key health problems affecting middle-aged and older adults. These conditions are long-lasting and often progress to cause irreversible damage. The prevalance of such conditions among the elderly is higher than among younger persons. The reported rates among the elderly for arthritis, heart conditions, hypertension, and vision and hearing impairments show the most substantial differences when compared with the prevalance rates of such chronic conditions among those under 65 years of age.

The presence of a chronic condition is often not as important to people as their consequent inability to carry out usual activities. However, just as the prevalence rates for chronic conditions increase with age, so does limitation of activity. Table 2.3 presents data on the self-reported health status of noninstitutionalized U.S. elderly by age and sex for the year 1976. The percentage of those unable to carry out a major activity, including working and keeping house, was considerably higher for men than women in both the young- and old-old groups. It is interesting that although females show higher prevalence rates for many chronic conditions, they report lower rates of major activity limitation than males. This may be due to the traditional social roles women have played which are less physically demanding than those of men. If this is the case, chronic conditions would be less likely to prevent women from meeting their obligations. Another possible explanation is that roles played by women (for example, wife, mother) are considered so essential that they must be carried out. Under such conditions, women (even older women) can ill afford to be reporting limitations in activity, even in the presence of chronic illness.

TABLE 2.3.   Self-reported health status of the noninstitutionalized elderly, by age and sex: 1976.

AGE	TOTAL	MEN	WOMEN
Percent Unable to Carry on Major Activity			
65 and over	17.6	29.9	9.0
65–74	14.7	26.6	5.5
75 and over	22.7	36.4	14.5
Percent Reporting Poor Health			
65 and over	9.0	9.3	8.8
65–74	8.5	9.2	8.1
75 and over	9.9	9.7	10.0

Source: Soldo, Beth J., "America's Elderly in the 1980's," *Population Bulletin,* Vol. 35, No. 4 (Population Reference Bureau, Inc., Washington, D.C., 1980).

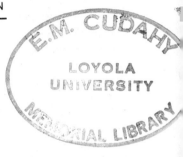

For all age and sex groups, the table shows no more than 10 percent of the elderly reporting themselves in poor health. Readers who are surprised at the relatively low percentages of the elderly reporting themselves to be in poor health or with major activity limitations may be manifesting a belief in one of the myths about aging, which is generally stated as follows: "A majority of old people have health problems." Apparently, the majority of older people *do not* have the kinds of health problems that limit their ability to work or keep house.

MARITAL STATUS AND LIVING ARRANGEMENTS

Table 2.4 presents a distribution of the population 65 years and over by marital status for both sexes for the years 1950 and 1975. The marital distribution of elderly men differs sharply from that of elderly women. In 1975, more than three out of four men were married and living with their

TABLE 2.4.   Distribution of the population 65 years old and over by marital status, males and females: 1950 and 1975.

MARITAL STATUS	MALES 1950	MALES 1975	FEMALES 1950	FEMALES 1975
Percent, Total	100.0	100.0	100.0	100.0
Single	8.0	4.7	8.0	5.8
Married	66.2	79.3	36.0	39.1
Spouse Present	63.3	77.3	34.3	37.6
Spouse Absent	2.9	2.0	1.7	1.5
Widowed	23.6	13.6	55.3	52.5
Divorced	2.2	2.5	0.7	2.6

Source: Siegel, J. *Demographic Aspects of Aging and the Older Population in the United States,* Current Population Reports, Special Studies, Series P-23 No. 59, May 1976.

wives; only 13.5 percent were widowed. Elderly women are much more likely to be widowed than married. In 1975, little more than a third of aged women (37.6 percent) were married and living with their husbands; *over one-half of all elderly women were widowed* (52.5 percent). As the table indicates, the changes in marital status from 1950 to 1975 have been quite substantial, especially for men. The proportion of elderly men who are married has increased while the proportion of single and widowed men has fallen significantly.

The two main factors that contribute to the different marital distributions of men and women are (1) the higher mortality rates of men (especially married men as compared with their wives) and (2) the higher remarriage rates of widowers. In the first instance, the expectation of life at age 65 of married women exceeds that of their husbands at age 70 by about nine years. Thus not only do most married women outlive their husbands, but they tend to do so by many years (Siegel, 1976). As for the second factor, the marriage rate for elderly men is about seven times that of elderly women and the vast majority of these are remarriages (Siegel, 1976).

There is also a difference in the household composition of elderly men and women. This very much reflects the differences in marital status between the sexes. Women are more than twice as likely to live alone as men (35.9 percent vs. 16.1 percent), while, as we have already seen, almost three-quarters of all men are married and living with their wives. The proportion of the elderly living alone appears to be increasing. This is chiefly the result of an increasing number of widows among the elderly and the improved economic situation of many elderly today over those in the past. Still, poverty as well as physical illness and disability remain two of the best reasons for living in a shared household.

GEOGRAPHIC
DISTRIBUTION

The elderly population, like the total population, is not distributed equally across the geographic terrain. Generally the elderly are numerically concentrated in the states that have the largest populations. In 1975, New York and California (with more than two million elderly each), Pennsylvania, Illinois, Ohio, Florida, and Texas accounted for 45.5 percent of the entire aged population of the United States. In 1979, the state with the highest percentage of elderly population was Florida (18.1), followed by Arkansas (13.7), Iowa and South Dakota (13.1 each), and Missouri and Nebraska (13.0). Less than three percent of Alaska's 1979 population was 65 years of age or older.

Increasingly, the elderly population has become an urban population. Only 27 percent of white elderly persons were located in rural areas of the United States in 1970 in contrast to 35 percent in 1950. The nonwhite elderly population is even more urban. Sections of many American cities can be characterized as "gray ghettos" (Cowgill, 1978), though this does not appear to result from any kind of intentional age segregation. According to Golant (1972), the growth of the urban elderly population is largely due to younger cohorts aging "in place" and residential relocations made earlier in the life cycle rather than after retirement.

Compared to younger persons, the elderly are much less likely to move. Among those who do move, some patterns are becoming evident. One need not be a professional demographer to recognize the elderly in-migration to states such as Florida and California. Out-migration is relatively high in the northeast and upper north-central region of the country.

According to Longino (1980), aged migrants move within the same general environmental settings—city dwellers move to cities, and residents of rural areas move to rural areas. This is the case even when migrants are changing states. In addition, Longino (1979) reports that a considerable proportion of interstate migrants are going "home." Among the older population, one-third of these migrants who resided outside of their state of birth in 1965 returned by 1970.

HOUSING
CHARACTERISTICS

Most Americans, including the elderly, live in single-family, owner-occupied homes. In 1973, about 73 percent of the elderly lived in their own homes compared to 65 percent of the non-elderly (Struyck and Soldo, 1980). Homes owned by the elderly were older than those owned by younger people. Almost

60 percent of elderly owner-occupants have lived in the same house since at least 1959 compared to only 19 percent of non-elderly owner-occupants. Thus it is not surprising to find that 62 percent of the homes owned and occupied by the elderly had been built before 1949 and that almost 75 percent of them had been built before 1940. Elderly renters also live in older structures. In 1976, almost one-half of the rental units occupied by the elderly were built before 1940.

The elderly live in household units that are somewhat more modest than those of the non-elderly. Among owner-occupants, the households are smaller by count of rooms and bathrooms, and have central heat less often. Among renters, smaller dwellings that are part of multiple unit (five or more) structures are utilized to a greater extent by the elderly than the non-elderly (Struyk and Soldo, 1980).

It is difficult to say whether the elderly live in less adequate housing than do the non-elderly. While some have offered poignant evidence of elderly persons living in dirty, unsafe and thoroughly wretched conditions, in general, defining what constitutes "adequate housing" has been problematic. There is no consensus on what measures should be included in such a standard. Struyk and Soldo (1980) used six indicators of housing inadequacy in their study of the quality of elderly housing. These included measures related to plumbing, kitchen facilities, sewage, heat, maintenance, and public halls. When compared with the non-elderly, the elderly were found to have a higher incidence of incomplete plumbing and kitchen facilities while both elderly and non-elderly households had a similar proportion of problems with the other measures of inadequacy.

A principal problem for the elderly is the large portion of their income that must be allocated to meet housing expenses. Struyk (1977) has suggested using a figure of 30 percent of total income devoted to housing as a criterion for excessive and burdensome housing cost. His analysis of the U.S. Bureau of the Census' Annual Housing Survey is that approximately 29 percent of all elderly households spend more than 30 percent of their income on housing. However, this figure is a composite of the wide variation that exists among different groups of the elderly. For example, 52 percent of those with incomes under $4,000, 50 percent of renters, and 44 percent of single persons spend more than 30 percent of their income on housing. With so many of the elderly choosing to spend a major share of their income on housing, an important question is whether sufficient income is available to purchase other needed goods and services (Struyk and Soldo, 1980).

EDUCATION

The extent of formal education received by older persons is considerably less than that of the general population. It is important to remember that people who are 75 years and older today grew up at a time when one-half of the

American population lived in rural areas, child labor was common, and few states had an adequate system of public high schools (Manard, Kart and van Gils, 1975). As table 2.5 shows, in 1970 the median years of school completed for this group was 8.5. Only about one-quarter (24.1) percent) of this population graduated from high school. This compares with a median of 10.6 years of school completed for those aged 55–64 years, 40.4 percent of whom were high school graduates.

TABLE 2.5   Educational status of the elderly, U.S., 1970, 2000.

AGE	1970	2000[1]
Median years of schooling completed		
55–64	10.6	12.5
65–74	8.8	12.3
75 +	8.5	12.1[2]
Percent of cohort that are high school graduates		
55–64	40.4	71.5
65–74	29.2	61.7
75 +	24.1	54.2[2]

[1]The projections for 2000 assume that no additional education is completed after 1970 and that differential mortality rates do not influence the measures of educational attainment for the cohort. Thus the estimates may somewhat underestimate the educational attainment of these cohorts in 2000.
[2]Only population aged 75–84 is represented in these figures.

Source: U.S. Bureau of the Census, *Census of Population: 1970 Subject Reports,* Final Report PC(2)-5B, "Educational Attainment," Washington, D.C.: U.S. Government Printing Office, 1973, Table 1.

In general, the level of education among the elderly population has been increasing. This reflects the movement of more educated, younger cohorts into the older age groups. By the year 2000, the United States Bureau of the Census projects that individuals aged 65–74 will have a median of 12.3 years of school completed and that over sixty percent (61.7 percent) of this population will have graduated from high school.

EMPLOYMENT

Older people have always worked. In fact, it was not until sometime between 1930 and 1940 that the rate of labor force participation by elderly American males dipped below 50 percent. This rate has continued to decline and by 1980 only about 20 percent of all elderly males were in the labor force. Among males aged 55-64 years (those approaching "normal" retirement age) labor force participation rates have declined only moderately during the twentieth century and are generally in line with overall employment trends among males. By 1947, 86.4 percent of all males 16 years of age and over were in the labor force. By 1974 this figure had dropped to 78.7 percent. The comparable figures for males aged 55-64 years were 89.6 percent and 77.4 percent respectively.

The percentage of women 65 years of age and over employed outside of the home has not exceeded 11 percent in this century. This low figure is surprising in light of the fact that the proportion of gainfully employed women of all ages has increased dramatically in the first three-quarters of the twentieth century. About 18 percent of all women were employed in 1890 and this figure has risen to over 45 percent in 1974. The labor force experience of women aged 55 to 64 reflects this phenomenon. Since 1947, labor force participation rates for this group have increased from 24.3 percent to 42 percent in 1979, though the rate peaked in 1970 (43 percent) and has shown minimal decline since.

What kind of work do older workers do? Historically, farming was the occupation in which most elderly men found work—it was a life-long occupation, as retirement on the farm was rare. An older farm worker physically unable to perform some duties could assume other less demanding but equally important chores. This was especially true for white farmers. A greater proportion of blacks than whites were in farming, but whites were much more likely to be owners or managers. Thus they were in position to remain in charge of planning and overseeing farm activities when they themselves were no longer able to carry out more physical farm duties.

As a source of jobs, farming has obviously diminished in importance—not just for older men, but for younger men as well. However, even in 1970 older workers of both sexes were more likely to be found in farming than were members of the general working population. As can be seen from Table 2.6, elderly male workers are almost three times as likely to be found in farm work than are all male workers (12.5 percent vs. 4.5 percent). Elderly females in the labor force are twice as likely to be in farm work as are female workers of all ages (1.4 percent vs. 0.7 percent).

Older workers are less likely than all workers to have blue-collar jobs. The reason for this is that many blue-collar jobs are in industries where mandatory retirement has been the rule and where pension plans are prevalent. Moreover, many blue-collar jobs are physically arduous—truck driving and construction work, for example.

Many older workers are self-employed or work for small businesses. These categories include accountants, lawyers, and tavern keepers who simply continue to work beyond age 65. Sales and clerical work are occupational categories ripe for part-time employment and, thus, amenable to elderly individuals attempting to supplement retirement; almost one-third (32.2 percent)

TABLE 2.6   Occupational distribution of employed persons: The total population and the elderly population, 1970.

	TOTAL POPULATION		POPULATION 65+	
	MALE	FEMALE	MALE	FEMALE
White Collar	*40.0%*	*61.6%*	*41.3%*	*53.1%*
Professional, technical and kindred	14.3	15.7	11.1	14.6
Managers and administrators (except farm)	11.2	3.6	12.9	6.3
Sales	6.9	7.4	10.1	10.7
Clerical and kindred	7.6	34.9	7.2	21.5
Blue Collar	*47.3%*	*17.2%*	*31.5%*	*14.0%*
Craftsmen and kindred	21.2	1.8	14.7	2.2
Operatives (except transport)	13.6	13.9	7.4	10.4
Transport equipment operatives	5.9	0.5	3.6	0.4
Laborers except farm	6.6	1.0	5.8	1.0
Farm	*4.5%*	*0.7%*	*12.5%*	*1.4%*
Farmers and farm managers	2.8	0.2	9.5	0.8
Farm laborers and foremen	1.7	0.5	3.0	0.6
Service	*8.1%*	*20.4%*	*14.8%*	*31.6%*
Service, except private households	8.1	16.6	14.5	18.1
Private household workers		3.8	0.3	13.5

Source: U.S. Department of Commerce, Bureau of Census, *Detailed Characteristics. United States Summary: 1970,* Table 226.

of all elderly female workers were employed in these categories in 1970.

Elderly workers are more likely than all workers to be found in service positions, having jobs as gardeners, seamstresses, practical nurses, washroom attendants, night watchmen, ticket takers, and domestics, among others. The 1970 Census reports relatively large proportions of elderly people in each of these occupations.

DOLLAR INCOME AND
ECONOMIC STATUS

Older Americans receive direct income from a variety of sources. Some have earnings from salaries, hourly wages, or from self-employment, while most have a retirement pension (including social security) of one kind or another. Other sources of direct monetary income are welfare payments, dividends, interest, rents, and alimony. Unemployment, veterans' and workmen's compensation payments, and gifts from others can also provide needed funds.

Figure 2.1 shows the sources of income for the elderly in 1976. Clearly, social security is the major source (39 percent), though earnings (23 percent) and asset income (18 percent) contribute to the income position of many of the elderly. Not all elderly individuals receive income from all the sources identified in Figure 2.1.

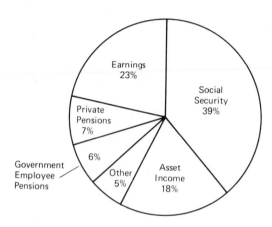

FIGURE 2.1.   Sources of Aged Income, 1976

Source: Grad, Susan and Karen Foster, *Income of the Population 65 and Older, 1976* (Washington, D.C.: Social Security Administration, 1979).

Just how much income do the elderly have? In 1977, most elderly persons had incomes under $6,000—this was the case for 55 percent of the men and 83 percent of the women. The median income of aged women was $3,088 while that of aged men was $5,526. This differential constitutes an income ratio of 55.8 percent. Only about 11 percent of aged men and 2 percent of aged women had incomes of $15,000 or more in 1977.

Another way of describing the income picture for the aged is in terms of family data. After all, many of the aged are married to someone who has income as well. Table 2.7 provides the median incomes of all families in America in 1977 including the median income for families in which the head of household is age 65 or over (hereafter referred to as "aged families"). The income of aged families is substantially higher than the income received by unrelated individuals, though it is still considerably below that of all families in the U.S. The median income of aged families in the U.S. in 1977 was $9,110, almost $7,000 less than the median for all families.

TABLE 2.7.   Median total money income by age of head of family, 1977.

		MEDIAN
Families		
	All ages	$16,009
	Head 65 years and over	9,110
Unrelated Individuals		
	All ages	5,907
	65 years and over	3,829

Source: U.S. Bureau of the Census, Consumer Income, Current Population Reports, Series P-60, No. 116 (Washington, D.C.: U.S. Government Printing Office, 1978).

Since 1965, the median income of aged families has increased more than two and one-half times, growing from $3,514 to $9,110. This change represents an increase of real income (above inflation) of approximately 40 percent. The relative income position of the aged also has shown improvement over the last dozen years. For example, the ratio of median income of aged families to the median income of all families rose from 49.3 percent in 1965 to 56.9 percent in 1977. However, this improvement in relative income status only reflects a return to the 1950 level of 57.3 percent (Clark, Kreps and Spengler, 1978).

It is important to remember that the elderly are a heterogeneous group and that there is a wide variation of income among them. We have already seen how income varies along the lines of sex and marital status. In addition, median income declines with age and income differences between those of the elderly who are working and those not working are substantial. In 1976, the median income of aged families where the head of household did not work was $7,850. In contrast, the median income of aged families headed by someone who worked full-time for more than 26 weeks in 1975 was approximately $16,000.

In 1968, the incidence of poverty among the elderly was about twice as great as the incidence of poverty in the total population. Table 2.8. shows that poverty declined among older people during the 1968–1977 period, though about one in seven older persons (14 percent) was still "officially" impoverished at the later date. Poverty varies among subgroups of the elderly. Aged whites are no more likely to live in poverty than anyone else in the U.S.—12 percent of this group live below the poverty level. However, 35 percent of their aged nonwhite counterparts are living in poverty.

TABLE 2.8.   Poverty rates: 1968, 1977.

	1968	1977
Total Population	13%	12%
Total Aged Population	25	14
Whites	23	12
Nonwhites	47	35

Source: Based on data in U.S. Bureau of the Census, *Consumer Income*, Current Population Reports, Series P-60, No. 116 (Washington, D.C.: U.S. Government Printing Office, 1978).

The above data on the poverty status of the elderly reflect the Social Security Administration's "poverty index," which is based on the amount of money needed to purchase a minimum adequate diet as determined by the Department of Agriculture. The index is calculated at three times the minimum adequate food budget (based on studies of consumers in 1955 and 1960–61) and varies by family size and composition with a farm/nonfarm differential for each family type. The index is not applied to the "hidden poor," those who are institutionalized or living with relatives. Thus, these figures on poverty status exclude more than one million aged who are unable to live independently.

Some argue that poverty is less acute among the elderly because of indirect or *in-kind income* they receive in the form of goods and services. According to the United States Select Committee on Aging (1979), there are 43 major federal programs benefiting the elderly in addition to those providing direct income. However, it is difficult to say how much income these programs provide to the aged. Measurement of indirect income is a problem because information on the value of comparable services available in the market place is sometimes difficult to obtain. In addition, the value which recipients may place on in-kind services may be quite different (more or less) than their actual market value (Schmundt, Smolensky, and Stiefel, 1975).

There are numerous programs aimed at providing housing for older people at a cost below that of similar housing on the open market. Under its various programs, the Department of Housing and Urban Development has rehoused approximately 750,000 older people, and about 600,000 of these people live in special housing for the elderly (Carp, 1976).

Perhaps the largest government program providing indirect income to the elderly is *Medicare*, the federal health insurance program for the aged, established in 1965. One example of how Medicare provides indirect income involves hospital care. In 1975, the total hospital bill for the elderly was $13.5 billion—Medicare paid for about 72 percent of this bill. Additional public monies paid for another 17.5 percent of this bill, leaving the remaining 10.5 percent or so being paid for by the particular elderly individual or some form of private health insurance.

The food stamp program is another visible source of indirect income to those of the elderly who are eligible to participate (there are income and assets requirements). In 1979, an aged couple with minimal assets (less than $3,000 excluding their home) and a gross annual income of $4,000 was eligible for coupons worth about $300 per year. The coupons can be used to purchase food in retail stores or, if the eligible person is disabled, to purchase prepared meals from specially designated programs.

The major direct income public welfare program for the elderly has been Old Age Assistance (OAA). Included in the Social Security Act of 1935 was a mandate for the establishment of a separate program of old-age assistance under which benefits (coming mostly from federal funds) would be distributed to the needy among the aged and be administered by the states. As a result of the states' administrative set-up, eligibility requirements and benefit levels varied considerably. Under the Social Security Amendments of 1972, a new federal program of *Supplemental Security Income* (SSI) for the aged, blind, and disabled replaced the former state-operated welfare program. This new program became effective on January 1, 1974.

The SSI program was envisioned as a basic national income maintenance system for the aged, blind, and disabled. It was intended to have minimal barriers to eligibility with lack of income being the principal requirement for participation. An individual's eligibility is determined by an "assets test" that is standardized nationally. The program was expected to supplement the social security program primarily by providing income support to those not covered by social security. Approximately two million aged individuals currently receive SSI benefits. As of January 1, 1983, SSI guarantees an income of $284.30 a month for an individual and $426.40 a month for a couple. This is still substantially below the poverty level, though many states provide an additional modest supplement to the federal benefit.

SUMMARY

The elderly population of the United States has increased eightfold since 1900. Changes in fertility, mortality and migration have all contributed to this growth. The absolute number of the elderly and the proportion of the population they constitute are expected to increase in this century, though at a slowed pace. However, the elderly population is still expected to number about 45 million by the year 2020, more than double the 1970 elderly population.

The old-age dependency ratio is a measure often used to summarize the demographic relationship between the elderly and the rest of the population. It is expected to increase in the coming years when a relatively smaller work force will be available to support a larger elderly population.

The aged population has become older during this century. The proportion of the aged who are 65–69 years of age has been and will continue to get smaller while the proportion of those 75 years of age and older has been getting larger—this trend is also expected to continue. Elderly women outnumber elderly men, a disparity that has been growing for the past several decades. Blacks constitute the largest group of nonwhite elderly, but, as a group, make up a smaller percentage of the total elderly population than they do the population at large.

Elderly women are much more likely to be widowed than married. In 1975, over one-half of all elderly women were widowed (52.5 percent). The marriage rate for elderly men is about seven times that of elderly women and the vast majority of these are remarriages. Consequently, elderly women are more than twice as likely to live alone as elderly men.

The elderly population is less residentially mobile than the younger population, though Florida and California show considerably higher rates of inmigration of the elderly than do the other states. Like the rest of the U.S. population, the elderly have become increasingly urbanized. Only about 25 percent of the total elderly population was located in rural America in 1970. Most elderly Americans live in single-family, owner-occupied homes. These households are, on the whole, somewhat more modest than those of the nonelderly, but it is difficult to say whether they are less than adequate. The principal problem for the elderly with regard to housing is that a sizable portion of income must be allocated to meet housing expenses.

Less than one-fourth of the aged male population is currently working. Many older workers are self-employed or work for small businesses. Elderly workers are more likely than all workers to be found in service jobs and less likely to be found in blue-collar work. Most elderly persons have incomes under $6,000. However, poverty has been declining among older people since the 1960s. About one in seven older persons (14 percent) is currently described by the federal government as being "officially" impoverished.

STUDY QUESTIONS

1. The elderly population has grown steadily during this century. Speculate about the probable growth rates of this population during the next fifty years. What are some considerations that could alter your predictions?

2. Distinguish between the "societal" old age dependency ratio and the "familial" old age dependency ratio.

3. What do the terms "young old and "old old" refer to in this text? How has the ratio between the two changed in this century?

4. Aged minority members are often described as being in "double jeopardy" in American society. What does this mean? Can you identify special problems faced by minority elderly?

5. Discuss the chief threats to the health status of older Americans. Do these threats differ by sex? How so?

6. Identify two factors that contribute to the different marital distribution between elderly men and women. Explain the changes in the marital distribution of elderly men that have occurred in the past twenty-five or thirty years.

7. What is a "gray ghetto?" Explain the concentration of the elderly in urban places in America. Describe the migration patterns of elderly Americans.

8. Identify some problems involved in determining the adequacy of housing for the elderly. What is the principal housing problem of the elderly in America?

9. What is the impact of age, work, and marital status on the income of elderly Americans?

BIBLIOGRAPHY

BUTLER, R., Why Survive? Being Old in America. New York, Harper & Row Pub., 1975.

CARP F., "Housing and Living Environments of Older People," in The Handbook of Aging and the Social Sciences, ed. by R. Binstock and E. Shanas. New York, Van Nostrand Reinhold, 1976.

CLARK, R., KREPS, J., and SPENGLER, J. "Economics of Aging: A Survey," Journal of Economic Literature, XVI (1978), 919–962.

COWGILL, D., "Residential Segregation by Age in American Metropolitan Areas," Journal of Gerontology, 33, 3(1978), 446–453.

CUTLER, N. and HAROOTYAN, R., "Demography of the Aged," in Aging: Scientific Perspectives and Social Issues, ed. by D. Woodruff and J. Birren. New York, D. Van Nostrand, 1975.

GOLANT, S., The Residential Location and Spatial Behavior of the Elderly. Chicago, Ill., University of Chicago, Department of Geography, Research Paper No. 143, 1972.

LONGINO, C., "Going Home: Aged Return Migration in the United States 1965-70," Journal of Gerontology, 34, 5(1979), 736–745.

———., "Residential Relocation of Older People: Metropolitan and Non-metropolitan," Research on Aging, 2, 2(1980), 205–16.

MANARD, B., KART, C., and VAN GILS, D., Old Age Institutions. Lexington, Mass., D.C. Health, Lexington Books, 1975.

NEUGARTEN, B., "The Future and the Young Old," Gerontologist, 15 (Part II), 1975, 4–9.

SCHMUNDT, M., SMOLENSKY, E., and STIEFEL, L., "The Evaluation of Recipients of In-Kind Transfers," in Integrating Income Maintenance Programs, ed. by I. Laurie. New York, Academic Press, 1975.

SIEGEL, J., Demographic Aspects of Aging and the Older Population in the United States. CPS, Special Studies, Series P-23, No. 59. Washington, D.C., U.S. Government Printing Office, 1976.

———, Prospective Trends in the Size and Structure of the Elderly Population, Impact of Mortality Trends, and Some Implications. CPS, Special Studies, Series P-23, No. 78. Washington, D.C., Bureau of the Census, 1979.

SOLDO, B., "America's Elderly in the 1980s," Population Bulletin, 35, 4(1980), 1–48.

STRUYK, R., "The Housing Expense Burden of Households Headed by the Elderly," *Gerontologist*, 17(1977), 447–452.

———and Soldo, B., *Improving the Elderly's Housing*. Cambridge, Mass., Ballinger, 1980.

TREAS, J., "Family Support Systems for the Aged: Some Social and Demographic Considerations." *Gerontologist*, 17, 6(1977), 486–491.

U.S. House Select Committee on Aging, *Federal Responsibility to the Elderly*. Washington, D.C., U.S. Government Printing Office, 1979.

CHAPTER THREE
ASSESSING THE
NUTRITIONAL STATUS
OF OLDER PEOPLE

Assessing the nutritional status of human beings is difficult. This is especially true in the United States because the population is so heterogeneous. Americans differ in racial and genetic background as well as in socioeconomic status in a way matched by few other nationalities. These variables have considerable impact on the form of an individual's nutritional intake. Another difficulty involves the various methods that can be used to assess nutritional status. In this chapter, for example (and thoughout the book, for that matter), the term "nutritional status" is sometimes used as if it had a uniform meaning. Careful readers will quickly become aware that this is not the case. As will be detailed below, nutritional status may refer to assessments made on the basis of measurements of dietary intake, biochemical tests, anthropometric and clinical findings, or any combination of these. In addition, it is fair to say that there is no consensus at present among nutritionists about the superiority of utilizing one combination of these methods over another for assessing nutritional status.

Nutritional status is an *operational term* that has to do with the way health is affected by food intake and the subsequent utilization of nutrients (Caliendo, 1979). What this means is that the research methods used, the specific responses measured, and the purposes of a particular study will determine the exact definition of nutritional status in that study. Additional confounding factors include whether the unit of measurement is an individual, a group (for example, the elderly), or a community (for example, Toledo, Ohio).

At first glance, the quantity of research on nutrition and old age appears to be abundant. Closer inspection, though, reveals that the quality of this research is inconsistent. Many studies are difficult to interpret because of small sample sizes, heterogeneity of subjects, and/or other questionable methodological considerations. However, some of the best available data has been collected on the general population in the United States and can be drawn upon to gain perspective on the nutritional problems of the aged (Barrows and Roeder, 1977).

Since 1936, in the United States, the Department of Agriculture (DOA) has at various times conducted studies on the dietary intake of Americans. The largest of these studies was carried out in 1965 and sampled almost 15,000 individuals from more than six thousand households. More recently, the U.S. Department of Health, Education and Welfare (now Health and Human Services), through the Center for Disease Control and the National Center for Health Statistics, has assessed the nutritional risk of groups of noninstitutionalized civilians. Two important surveys carried out by this department are the Ten-State Nutrition Survey conducted between 1968 and 1970 and the so-called HANES (Health and Nutrition Examination Survey) carried out in 1971–72. These studies were not specifically designed to gather data on aged people, but each includes substantial samples of older Americans. We begin this chapter by describing these three important national surveys and summarizing the findings on the relationship between age and nutritional status.

NATIONAL SURVEYS

Household Food Consumption Survey, 1965–66

This nationwide study, carried out by the U.S. Department of Agriculture, was intended to assess the nutritional status of the general population in the United States. One component of the survey asked for and obtained information on the food intake for one day of a representative sample of 14,519 men, women, and children from over six thousand households. This was the first time nationwide estimates of the food eaten in a 24-hour period by individuals became available. Principal objectives of the survey included determining the nutritive value of the food intake of individuals at different stages of the life cycle as well as enumeration of which sex-age groups used vitamin and/or mineral supplements.

We will concern ourselves here with those findings reported from the one-day survey which are relevant to describing the nutritional situation of older Americans. The survey did not include individuals living in institutions or group quarters such as rooming houses. Thus some aged individuals, perhaps those most likely to be ill or disabled, were omitted from the survey. In addition, approximately two-thirds of all the individuals surveyed were from the urban North. Also, considerably more older persons were members of households with low incomes than were younger adults included in the survey. Among those surveyed, almost one-half (48 percent) of all adults 65 years and over were in households with a 1964 family income, after taxes, of under $3,000. In contrast, only 13 percent of all adults under 65 years of age had this level of income. Only nine percent of the elderly, as opposed to 26 percent of those under 65 years of age, were in households with incomes of $8,000 and over.

For most foods of all categories, the survey reports that consumption peaked (especially for males) in the late teens and early adulthood. There was less difference by age in the amounts of food eaten by females than by males. There was also less difference among age groups in the consumption of fruits and vegetables than in the consumption of higher calorie foods. The average diets for most sex-age groups approached 90 to 100 percent (or more) of the Recommended Dietary Allowances (RDAs) set by the Food and Nutrition Board of the National Academy of Sciences–National Research Council in 1968 for energy, protein, vitamin A value, thiamine, riboflavin, and ascorbic acid. Calcium and iron were the nutrients most often found below allowances.

In general, the diets of older men met the standards for RDAs for more nutrients than the diets of older women. As Table 3.1 shows, men aged 55 to 74 had diets low in calcium, while those 75 and over showed deficiencies in calcium, vitamin A, riboflavin, and ascorbic acid. Older women were below the RDAs in their intake of calcium, iron, vitamin A, thiamine, and riboflavin. Survey data also show the aged far below the recommended allowances for vitamin B_6 and magnesium, though recommended levels of vitamin B_6, vitamin B_{12}, and magnesium appear to be difficult to meet for adults of all ages.

Perhaps the most important finding in the Household Food Consumption Survey has to do with the relationship between income and dietary adequacy (based on achieving RDAs). Almost two-thirds (63 percent) of those with incomes, after taxes, of less than $3,000 were found to have less than adequate diets. The nutrients most often below RDAs for the poor were ascorbic acid, vitamin A, calcium, and iron. Finally, older people were found to be high-frequency users of mineral or vitamin supplements. About one-third of those 75 years of age and over used such supplements, but even here the use of such supplements was found to increase with income.

Ten-State Nutrition Survey, 1968-70

The Ten-State Nutrition Survey was the first comprehensive survey ever developed to assess the problems of serious hunger and malnutrition involving a large segment of the population of the United States. Groups suspected of being at high risk for malnutrition were intentionally overreprepresented in this study. These included the poor, migrant groups, the Spanish-speaking

TABLE 3.1.   Nutrient intake below recommended allowance, Household Food Consumption Survey, U.S., 1965–66.

SEX-AGE (YEARS)	PROTEIN	CALCIUM	IRON	VITAMIN A VALUE	THIAMINE	RIBO-FLAVIN	ASCORBIC ACID
Male:							
55–64		**					
65–74		**					
75 and over		***		*		**	*
Female:							
55–64		****			*	*	
65–74		****	*	*	**	**	
75 and over		****	*	**	**	***	

Below by: * 1–10%   ** 11–20%   *** 21–29%   **** 30% or more
Average intake of group below Recommended Dietary Allowance, NAS-NRC, 1968. U.S. diets of men, women, and children, 1 day in Spring 1965.

Source: U.S. Department of Agriculture, Agricultural Research Service. *Household Food Consumption Survey, 1965-66, Report II, Food and Nutrient Intake of Individuals in the United States, Spring 1965.* Washington, D.C.: U.S. Government Printing Office.

population in the southwest, people living in the inner cities, and individuals living in industrial areas where a significant work force had moved in from the South during the previous 10 to 20 years. While geographical disparity was a concern, more important was the inclusion of geographical areas assumed to contain the targeted populations. Ten states were selected: Texas, Louisiana, Kentucky, Michigan, New York (including a separate survey of New York City), Massachusetts, Washington, California, West Virginia, and South Carolina. The sample was drawn from 1960 Census enumeration districts where the largest percentage of families were living in poverty. Because of changes in residential patterns between 1960 and the time the surveys were actually carried out in the different states (1968–70), middle- and upper-income individuals were also included. Nearly 24,000 families took part in the Ten-State Nutrition Survey—a total of 86,352 persons—making this the largest study of its kind ever conducted.

The following basic measurements were incorporated into the plan of the study: (1) clinical assessments including medical history; (2) physical examinations and various anthropometric measurements; (3) biochemical measurements of the levels of various substances in blood and urine; (4) dietary assessment of nutrient intake and usual patterns of food consumption; (5) dental examinations; and (6) related sociodemographic data.

Generally, persons 60 years of age and older were found to consume far less food than needed to meet the nutrient standards for their age, sex, and weight. A comparison made with the same age group surveyed in the 1965 USDA study (referred to above) showed only minor differences in eating habits, though mean intakes of calories and nutrients for participants in Ten-State Survey were generally lower than those for persons in the USDA survey. (See Table 3.2.)

While diets of the elderly were lower in calories than diets of younger persons, the Ten-State Survey found the former to be of higher quality based on nutrient intake per 1000 calories. This was particularly true for protein, iron, vitamin A, and for vitamin C in females. Diet quality did not vary across subgroups, with the exception of vitamin A intake. Blacks showed very high intakes of vitamin A while Spanish-Americans had very low intakes.

In the process of investigating the relationship between income and dietary intake, Ten-State Survey researchers employed a measure referred to as a "Poverty Income Ratio" (PIR). Each family in the study received a weighted PIR value based on income, family composition, household size, sex of the head of household, and whether a farm or nonfarm residence was being considered. A family with a PIR of 1.0 was considered to be living at the poverty level. Ratios of less than 1.0 can be referred to as "below poverty"; ratios greater than 1.0 as "above poverty." In addition, both mean and median values for PIR were computed for each state. A state was designated as "low-income-ratio" if it had a median PIR below 1.39, the median poverty income ratio for all families in all states for whom income data were avail-

TABLE 3.2. Mean nutrient intake of all persons sixty years of age and over in the Ten-State Survey compared with the nutritive value of diets of persons sixty-five through seventy-four years of age in the United States Department of Agriculture Survey (Spring 1965) by sex.

	NUMBER OF PERSONS	CALORIES	MEAN NUTRIENT INTAKE							
			PROTEIN (GM)	CALCIUM (MG)	IRON (MG)	VITAMIN A (I.U.)	THIAMINE (MG)	RIBO-FLAVIN (MG)	PREFORMED NIACIN (MG)	VITAMIN C (MG)
Male										
Ten-State Nutrition Survey..........	895	1949	80.1	736	13.1	4979	1.14	1.76	19.06	59
U.S.D.A 1965	460	2058	82.5	691	13.5	5800	1.17	1.70	N.A.	66
Female										
Ten-State Nutrition Survey..........	1233	1412	59.5	568	9.6	5172	0.86	1.40	14.72	67
U.S.D.A. 1965	624	1473	60.3	502	9.8	4940	0.84	1.25	N.A.	57

N.A.: Not Available

Source: U.S. Department of Health, Education and Welfare. Ten-State Nutrition Survey, 1968–70, Vol. V—Dietary. Pub. No. (HSM) 72–8133. Atlanta, Ga.: Center for Disease Control, p. 267, Table 3.

able. This group of states included South Carolina, Louisiana, Texas, Kentucky, and West Virginia. States with a median PIR equal to or greater than 1.39 were labelled "high-income-ratio" and included Michigan, California, Washington, Massachusetts, and New York.

Figure 3.1 shows the average caloric intake of specific PIR groups for the low and high income ratio states. While the differences were not substantial, each PIR group that included persons from high income ratio states showed higher average caloric intake. However, the relationship between PIR and nutrient intake per 1000 calories is still inconsistent. Table 3.3 presents data on nutrient intake per 1000 calories for aged males only, by PIR group for both low and high income ratio states. When compared with those residing in high income ratio states (PIR of 1.00 or more), individuals residing in low income ratio states (PIR less than 1.00) show higher intake of calcium, vitamin A, thiamine, riboflavin, and vitamin C, and lower intake of protein, iron, and niacin.

The clinical assessment of adults contained in the Ten-State Survey presented little evidence of malnutrition in the population examined. It appears that the value of clinical examination is yet to be determined, especially in the assessment of less-than-obvious malnutrition (U.S. Department of Health, Education and Welfare, 1975). Anthropometric measurements in the Survey included height, weight, skeletal mass, and obesity. Skeletal weight appears to decline after age 50, reflecting an increasing loss and porosity of

FIGURE 3.1.   Mean caloric intake per kilogram of body weight for all persons sixty years of age and over by specified poverty income ratio groups for low income ratio states and high income ratio states—Ten-State Nutrition Survey (1968–70). (Source: U.S. Department of Health, Education and Welfare. *Ten-State Nutrition Survey, 1968–70, Vol. V—Dietary.* Pub. No. HSM 72-8133. Atlanta, Ga.: Center for Disease Control, p. 269, Figure 2.)

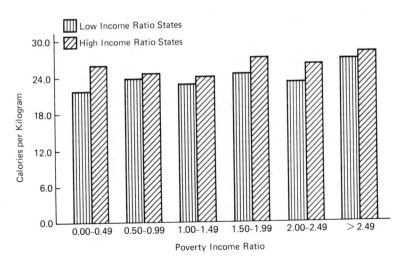

TABLE 3.3. Mean nutrient intake per 1000 calories of selected nutrients for males sixty years of age and over by specified poverty income ratio groups for low income ratio states and high income ratio states — Ten-State Nutrition Survey (1968–1970).

POVERTY INCOME RATIO GROUP	NUMBER OF PERSONS	MEAN CALORIC INTAKE	MEAN NUTRIENT INTAKE PER 1000 CALORIES							
			PROTEIN (GM)	CALCIUM (MG)	IRON (MG)	VITAMIN A (I.U.)	THIAMINE (MG)	RIBO-FLAVIN (MG)	PREFORMED NIACIN (MG)	VITAMIN C (MG)
LOW INCOME RATIO STATES										
Less than 1.00	535	1446	39.54	412.67	6.57	3472.81	0.66	0.99	9.12	41.76
1.00 or greater	242	1611	44.44	409.74	6.98	3000.39	0.62	1.03	9.88	37.75
HIGH INCOME RATIO STATES										
Less than 1.00	300	1615	42.69	426.46	7.54	2300.00	0.63	0.92	10.59	38.43
1.00 or greater	741	1796	41.66	371.32	6.66	3134.00	0.55	0.90	10.48	38.29

Note: Dietary data presented in this table are based on twenty-four hour recall.

Source: U.S. Department of Health, Education and Welfare. Ten-State Nutrition Survey, 1968–70, Vol. V—Dietary. Pub. No. (HSM) 72-8133. Atlanta, Ga.: Center for Disease Control, p. 269, Table 6.

bone that is comparable in both the high and low PIR groups. Older black women show the highest prevalence of obesity—over 50 percent in the 45- to 55-year-old age group and over 45 percent in the 55- to 65-year-old group. More than one-third of all white women in the 55- to 65-year-old group were defined as obese in the Ten-State Survey. Among the elderly, the lowest prevalence of obesity was found in black males. The relationship between income level and obesity is clear for males of both races, but for females income was not consistently associated with the prevalence of obesity. Higher income level was associated with a higher prevalence of obesity in both black and white males.

Periodontal disease was discovered to be a major problem in adults over 35 years of age. Its prevalence increased with age to over a 90 percent occurrence in nearly every subgroup of the survey population by the age of 65–75 years. Scores on a Periodontal Index (PI) were slightly lower (indicating clinical health) in high income ratio states than in low income ratio states, yet in both categories of states, PI scores increased with age (indicating periodontal disease). Taken as a whole, the data generally show poor dental health to be associated with poor levels of dental care in the population surveyed, not malnutrition.

Biochemical measures of nutritional status did not suggest that particular deficiencies were associated with age. For example, while the Survey revealed relatively low hemoglobin values in the older population, there was a high prevalence of such values in all population subgroups, particularly among blacks. Along with the findings of lower-than-recommended iron intakes for selected subgroups of the population, the Ten-State Survey identified nutritional iron deficiency as a national public health problem.

Health and Nutrition Examination Survey, 1971–72 (HANES)

The HANES program was undertaken by the National Center for Health Statistics to establish a continuing national nutrition survey under the authority of the National Health Survey Act of 1956. Preliminary findings are available from the first examination of 10,126 persons ages 1–74 years drawn from a representative subset of 35 of 65 primary sampling units identified by the U.S. Bureau of the Census. Data was collected between April 1971 and October 1972, and researchers with the National Center for Health Statistics believe the resulting observations to be "much more closely representative of the civilian noninstitutionalized population of the United States than estimates from any previous survey on nutrition."

The HANES was designed to provide data to assess the adequacy of nutrient intake of Americans. The specific measurement methods employed in HANES, which were similar to those used in the Ten-State Survey, included information on dietary intake, biochemical tests (including blood and urinalysis), clinical examination, and anthropometric measurements. One important difference between the Ten-State Survey and HANES involves the evaluation of dietary intake. The set of standards employed for the evaluation of the HANES dietary data was developed using the recommendations of an *ad hoc* advisory group that considered standards from a variety of organizations including the World Health Organization and the National Research Council Food and Nutrition Board Recommended Dietary Allowances. Table 3.4 shows these standards for persons 60 years of age and older by sex.

TABLE 3.4.   Standards for evaluation of daily dietary intake used in the HANES, 1971-72: Persons 60 years of age and older.

	MALE	FEMALE
Calories (per kg)	34	29
Protein (gm per kg)	1.0	1.0
Calcium (mg)	400	600
Iron (mg)	10	10
Vitamin A (I.U.)	3500	3500
Vitamin C (mg)	60	55

Source: National Center for Health Statistics, *Preliminary Findings of the First Health and Nutrition Examination Survey, United States, 1971-72: Dietary Intake and Biochemical Findings.* DHEW Publication No. (HRA) 74-1219-1, Health Resources Administration. Washington, D.C., Government Printing Office.

The data for those aged 60 and over were presented according to race and income status. Two income groups were used: (1) income below poverty level, indicated by a PIR (the same measure employed in the Ten-State Survey) of less than one; and (2) income at and above the poverty level, indicated by a PIR of 1.00 or more. A substantial proportion of all persons age 60 and over had low daily caloric intake. Among those with low income, 27 percent of the white and 36 percent of the black aged had caloric intakes of less than 1,000 calories. The corresponding figures for those in the income group above the poverty level were 16 and 18 percent respectively. Protein intake was also related to income in this age group. Both blacks and whites in the higher income group had higher mean intakes of protein than those in the lower income group. However, mean protein intakes per 1,000 calories showed little or no variation by race or income, suggesting that protein consumption was closely related to total caloric intake.

Intake for other nutrients (calcium, iron, vitamins A and C) must be looked at closely for those age 60 and over. A cursory inspection of data appears to show that all race and income status groupings have an average intake of these four nutrients in excess of 100 percent of the standard. Only those with income below poverty level (both white and black) showed mean iron intake below 100 percent of the standard and these values were 95 and 93 percent respectively. However, more careful inspection, as given in Table 3.5, indicates that substantial proportions of all race and income groups have daily nutrient intakes below the standard.

TABLE 3.5.   Percentage below standard daily nutrient intake values for persons aged 60 and over by race for income levels: United States, 1971-72 (HANES).

NUTRIENT	TOTAL	WHITE		BLACK	
		INCOME BELOW POVERTY LEVEL	INCOME ABOVE POVERTY LEVEL	INCOME BELOW POVERTY LEVEL	INCOME ABOVE POVERTY LEVEL
Calcium[1]	37%	40%	34%	45%	47%
Iron	50	63	47	67	65
Vitamin A	56	61	56	62	52
Vitamin C[2]	39	56	37	55	43

[1]The lower standard of 400 mg for men is used.
[2]The lower standard of 55 mg for females is used.
Source: National Center for Health Statistics, *Preliminary Findings of the First Health and Nutrition Examination Survey, United States, 1971-72: Dietary intake and Biochemical Findings.* DHEW Publication No. (HRA) 74-1219-1, Health Resources Administration. Washington, D.C., Government Printing Office.

The table shows that iron and vitamin A intakes were less than the standards for more than 50 percent of all persons over 60 with the exception of whites with income above the poverty level—47 percent of the latter group had iron intakes below the daily standard. For blacks, income seemed to affect daily intake of vitamins A and C. For example, 55 percent of blacks who had income below the poverty level also were below the standard for daily intake of vitamin C—this compares with 43 percent of blacks above the poverty income level. For whites, income had a similar impact on iron and vitamin C intake. Whites with income below the poverty level were much more likely to have a substandard intake of iron than those above it (63 and 47 percent respectively). Vitamin C intake was also more likely to be deficient in the former group than in the latter (56 and 37 percent).

Biochemical tests revealed little about nutritional problems among the elderly in the HANES data. Low income blacks had the highest incidence of low hemoglobin and hematocrit values of any aged group. This group also shows very low percentages of low serum irons and percent transferrin saturation, which is not readily explainable if iron deficiency is excluded as a cause. Aged blacks had the highest mean serum proteins of all subgroups (with the lowest percent of low values), though this too remains without explanation.

Anthropometric and clinical findings from HANES have only recently become available. Obesity, measured by triceps skinfold thickness, shows a pattern similar to that reported in the Ten-State Survey. Older black women had the highest prevalence of obesity (32.4 percent in the 45–74 age group), with the lowest prevalence found in older black men (7.7 percent in the 45–74 age group). Lower income was more consistently associated with a higher prevalence of obesity among women than men.

Table 3.6 summarizes the preliminary findings for persons aged 60 years and over by race and income level. In general, the clinical data show a very low percentage of high and moderate risk signs for most nutritional deficiencies. There are several exceptions in which the percent prevalence does exceed ten percent. These include a moderate risk of niacin deficiency for all aged, clinically signaled by fissures of the tongue, and a moderate risk of thiamine deficiency among aged blacks, reflected in a high prevalence rate of absent ankle jerks. A low risk of vitamin C deficiency appears to exist for all of the aged, excepting blacks, who may exhibit two clinical signs of deficiency.

The national surveys summarized above indicate that a substantial proportion of the U.S. aged population is nutritionally vulnerable. A large number of the aged consume diets that are insufficient in calories and deficient in nutrients necessary for maintaining physical health and well-being. Those particularly vulnerable would seem to be the low-income aged and those who are sick or disabled. While the surveys excluded the institutionalized and did not evaluate the general health status of respondents, it is well known that disease weighs heavily on the maintenance of adequate nutritional status. The national surveys also show that many of the aged are consuming diets wholly inappropriate as therapeutic regimens for managing acute or chronic diseases. Similar conclusions were reached by Watkin (1968), who indicated that nutritional status of the elderly was more related to income and health status than to age per se.

LOCAL AND REGIONAL STUDIES

Numerous local and regional nutrition studies have been carried out using a variety of elderly subject populations. Table 3.7 summarizes 25 different studies of dietary intake and is organized into three basic methodological caterogies: recalls, food records, and dietary histories. The table includes information on the location of the study, the number, sex and age of the subject population, housing arrangements, the number of nutrients for which diets were analyzed, and the purpose of carrying out the study. Later in this chapter, the problems involved in doing research on the nutritional status of older persons will be discussed and will include the advantages and disadvantages of various techniques. Here we wish to describe the results of several often-cited local studies represented in the table in order to shed additional light on the factors which may predispose the elderly to nutritional problems.

Lebovit (1965) examined the dietary intake of members of 283 Rochester households. Data were collected by personal interview, using the "recall" method, and information on food used was taken for the week immediately preceding the interview. All interviewees lived alone or with someone 55 years of age or older and all were Social Security recipients. They generally had low income levels, and received little formal schooling. Forty percent were immigrants and 25 percent were first generation Americans. They owned their own homes and ate most meals at home. Eighty percent of the households had food supplies that met the full 1963 Recommended Dietary Allowances (RDAs) for thiamine, protein, iron, vitamin A, riboflavin, and calories. Seventy percent met the RDAs for calcium and ascorbic acid, though it is these two that the study found in short supply in diets. What the respondents ate is another matter. Only about 50 percent had diets that provided the nutrient allowances in full. Twenty-five percent of the households had diets that met two-thirds of the allowances for all nutrients. Diets of a quarter of the households were below two-thirds of the RDAs for one or more nutrients. The "poorest" diets were found among men living alone, the oldest (those 75 years or older), those with lowest incomes, and those spending less on food than the money value of the U.S. Department of Agriculture's low-cost diet plan. Interestingly, there was no relationship between health problems and the nutritive quality of diets. Some evidence in the study suggests that those with less motivation or interest in food made the poorest food supply and dietary choices.

Fry and her coworkers (1963) used weighed intakes (for periods ranging from 25 to 120 days) and seven-day dietary records to determine the intake of a small sample of elderly, healthy, and community-active women in Nebraska. Average daily intake of calories and all nutrients, except iron, either met or exceeded the recommended daily allowances. In addition to iron, intake of calcium and vitamin A were consumed at less than satisfactory levels in the diets of a small percentage of these women. Approximately one-half of the average caloric intake of the women sampled was provided by fat, while one-third was provided by carbohydrates. The authors believe that this pattern of nutrient intake may represent a geographical phenomenon. They cite one study which suggests that women in the North Central states eat appreciably more fat than California women. To the extent that dietary fat has been implicated in the development of atherosclerosis and heart disease, this should be of some concern. Finally, this study found significant variation in calories and nutrient intake over time in the diets of some sample members. The particular dietary pattern of the individual seems more important in explaining this variation than methodological concerns such as the length of

TABLE 3.6. Clinical findings for persons aged 60 years and over by race and income level: number of persons and percent with positive clinical signs suggestive of specific nutrient deficiency by risk category, United States, 1971–72 (HANES Preliminary).

NUTRIENT DEFICIENCY AND CLINICAL SIGNS BY RISK CATEGORY	ALL INCOME			INCOME BELOW POVERTY LEVEL[2]			INCOME ABOVE POVERTY LEVEL[2]		
	TOTAL[1]	WHITE	BLACK	TOTAL[1]	WHITE	BLACK	TOTAL[1]	WHITE	BLACK
n (examined persons)	1,938	1,486	435	484	292	191	1,331	1,104	212
N (estimated population in thousands)	20,560	18,719	1,791	3,113	2,397	714	15,949	14,996	906
Protein									
Hepatomegaly (M)	4.0	4.2	2.3	2.5	2.5	2.8	4.2	4.4	1.8
Potbelly (M)	-	-	-	-	-	-	-	-	-
Riboflavin									
Magenta tongue (H)	0.0	0.0	-	0.0	1.0	-	0.0	0.0	-
Angular lesions of lips (H)	1.2	1.3	-	1.8	2.4	-	1.1	1.1	-
Angular scars of lips (H)	0.0	0.0	0.0	0.0	-	-	0.0	0.0	0.0
Nasolabial seborrhea (M)	0.0	0.0	0.0	1.0	1.0	0.0	0.0	0.0	0.0
Conjunctival injection (L)	1.0	1.0	0.0	1.0	1.0	0.0	1.0	1.0	0.0
Niacin									
Filiform papillary atrophy of tongue (H)	4.9	4.8	6.1	3.4	3.0	4.6	5.4	5.3	8.4
Scarlet beefy tongue (H)	1.0	1.0	0.0	3.2	4.2	-	1.0	1.0	-
Fungiform papillary hypertrophy of tongue (M)	1.7	1.6	2.8	2.6	2.0	4.7	1.6	1.6	1.4
Fissures of tongue (M)	13.2	13.1	14.6	11.9	11.8	12.2	13.3	13.0	18.2
Serrations or swelling of tongue (L)	6.1	6.4	3.3	7.7	8.4	5.3	5.4	5.7	2.3

Thiamine									
Absent knee jerks (M)	2.3	1.9	5.8	3.6	3.7	3.4	2.1	1.8	7.7
Absent ankle jerks (M)	7.1	6.5	13.6	7.7	4.9	17.3	6.7	6.4	12.2
Vitamin D									
Bowed legs (M)	5.4	5.5	4.3	8.2	8.8	6.4	5.0	5.1	2.8
Knock knees (M)	1.0	1.0	2.5	1.7	1.5	2.4	1.0	1.0	2.7
Vitamin A and/or essential fatty acid									
Follicular hyperkeratosis, arms (M)	2.2	1.9	5.6	2.4	2.3	2.7	2.4	2.0	8.9
Follicular hyperkeratosis of upper back (L)	0.0	0.0	0.0	-	-	-	0.0	0.0	-
Dry or scaling skin (L)	9.2	9.4	7.4	7.2	7.4	6.7	9.6	9.8	6.9
Vitamin C									
Bleeding and swollen gums (M)	4.0	3.7	6.7	9.2	9.5	8.5	3.2	3.0	5.4
Swollen red papillae (L)	7.3	5.6	23.6	15.6	8.5	31.9	6.1	5.6	15.4
Diffuse Marginal inflammation (L)	26.6	23.7	52.7	53.8	44.5	75.1	22.2	21.2	37.4
Iodine									
Thyroid enlargement									
Group I (M)	2.6	2.6	2.6	3.1	2.7	4.4	2.8	2.8	1.4
Group II (H)	1.1	1.0	3.2	1.2	1.1	1.6	1.1	1.0	5.0
Calcium									
Positive Chvostek's sign (M)	1.3	1.2	2.8	1.8	1.7	2.1	1.3	1.2	3.9

[1]Total includes all races.
[2]Excludes persons with unknown income.

(H) = high risk indicator of possible deficiency;
(M) = moderate risk indicator of possible deficiency;
(L) = low risk indicator of possible deficiency.

Source: National Center for Health Statistics, *Preliminary Findings of the First Health and Nutrition Examination Survey, United States, 1971–72: Anthropometric and Clinical Findings.* DHEW Publication No. (HRA) 75–1229, Health Resources Administration. Washington, D.C., Government Printing Office.

TABLE 3.7. Description of studies of nutrition and aging.

FIRST AUTHOR	LOCATION	SUBJECTS NO.	SEX	AGE	HOUSING	DIETARY METHODOLOGY	NO. NUTRIENTS ANALYZED	PURPOSE
Todhunter	Middle Tenn.	343 / 186	F / M	60+ / 60+	Free-living	24-hr recall	7	To determine nutritive adequacy of meals and reasons for any inadequacies
Goodman	Luzerne County, Pa.	389 / 184	F / M	60+ / 60+	Free-Living	24-hr recall	8	To assess impact of congregate meals program for elderly; to test validity of 24-hr recall when used with elderly persons
Guthrie	Rural Pennsylvania	40 / 69	M / F	>60 / >60	Own homes and apartments	24-hr recall	8	To evaluate nutritional adequacy of elderly rural citizens
Joering	Cinn., Ohio	135 / 50	F / M	45–90 / 45–90	Own homes or apartments	24-hr recall	9	To determine nutritional contribution of meal program to dietary needs of senior citizens
Nutrition Canada	Ten provinces, reserves, and crownlands	GENERAL POPULATION 926 / 859; INDIANS 116 / 114; ESKIMOS 29 / 19	M / F; M / F; M / F	65+ / 65+; 55+ / 55+; 55+ / 55+	Free-living	24-hr recall	8	To determine nutritional status of the Canadian population

Investigator	Location	Sex	No.	Age	Setting	Method	No.	Purpose
Lebovit	Rochester, N.Y.	M	179	avg 74	Free-living	1-wk recall	8	To learn more about dietary problems of the aging
		F	277	avg 71				
Davidson	Boston, Mass.	M	42	65+ 51-97	Own homes and apartments	1-wk recall plus 1-wk food records	9	To determine relationship of nutrient intake to various social and economic variables
		F	62	51-97				

Food records (1 to 4 days)

Investigator	Location	Sex	No.	Age	Setting	Method	No.	Purpose
Kohrs	Central Mo.	M	149	59-96	Free-living	1-day food records	9	To evaluate effect of meals program on adequacy of nutrient intake of older Americans
		F	317	59-96				
Greger	Indianapolis, Ind.	M	18	52-89	Free-living	1-day food record cross-checked by recall	15	To assess adequacy of zinc intake through analysis of hair and determination of taste acuity; to estimate dietary intake of title VII feeding program participants
		F	26	52-89				
Steinkamp	Berkeley, Calif.	1962 STUDY						To relate nutritional status to mortality rate; to determine nutritional status and dietary habits over 14-yr period
		M	98	64-98	Free-living	1-day food records	9	
		F	131	64-98				
		4 STUDY YEARS						
		M	68					
		F	73					
Hankin	Milwaukee, Wis.	M	23	>60	Nursing home	3-day food record (also 1-wk inventory of 13 nursing homes)	5	To determine if sufficient food purchased to meet RDA and if individual meals of selected patients provide adequate nutrients
		F	42	>60				

TABLE 3.7. (Continued)

FIRST AUTHOR	LOCATION	SUBJECTS NO.	SUBJECTS SEX	SUBJECTS AGE	HOUSING	DIETARY METHODOLOGY	NO. NUTRIENTS ANALYZED	PURPOSE
Food records (over 4 days)								
Justice	West Lafayette, Ind.	12 32	M F	63–93 63–93	Nursing home	5 or 6 nonconsecutive days of food records recorded by a dietitian	13	To determine differences in status found in elderly ill requiring extended nursing care
Dibble	Syracuse, N.Y.	33 67	M F	50+ 50+	Free-living in public senior housing	6-day food records	7	Information on nutrient intake and status of healthy persons living in own household, alone or with spouse
McGandy	Baltimore, Md., and Washington, D.C.	252 (137 were	M	20–99 55+)	Free-living	7-day food records	9	To evaluate effect of age on dietary intake; to estimate energy expenditure and its relation to caloric intake at various ages
Fry	Lincoln, Nebr.	26	F	65–85	Own home	7-day food records (plus weighed intake 25–120 days for 6)	11	To determine the intake of nutrients of active, healthy women 65 yr or older
Davidson	Boston, Mass.	42 62	M F	51–97 51–97	Own home or apartment	1-wk food record (also 1-wk recall)	9	To determine nutrient intake and its relation to social and economic variables
Weighed intake								
Harrill	Fort Collins and Denver, Colo.	15 45	F F	65+ 65+	Own home Nursing home	3-day weighed intake	8	To compare the nutrient intake of institutionalized and free-living women
Fry	Lincoln, Nebr.	6	F	68–80	Own home	Weighed intake 25–120 days (also 26 7-day records)	11	To determine intake of nutrients of active healthy women 65 years or older

Investigator	Location	No.	Sex	Age	Setting	Method	No.	Purpose
Tucker	Rhode Island	24 24	M F	60 60	Ambulatory residents of public institution for aged	14-day weighed food records	9	To study intake of individuals residing in institution for aged in comparison to RDA and to average portion served in institution
Ohlson	Lansing, Mich.	18	F	48–77	Free-living	Weighed diet 3–4 mo. Also balance study 10 days each month	3	To determine nitrogen, calcium, and phosphorus retention of older women
Dietary histories								
Clarke	Within 75 miles of Manhattan, Kansas	99 98	M and F M and F	70+ 70+	Nursing home Independent housing	Food frequency questionnaire: 22 food groups, trained interviewers	8	To compare eating behavior of nursing home residents to elderly living in own home
Kohrs	Missouri	45 66	M F	59+ 59+	Free-living	Dietary history	9	Subgroup of large survey to determine the nutritional status of Missouri residents
Lyons	Boston, Mass.	30 70	M F	65+ 65+	Free-living	Dietary history	9	To study nutritional status and health status of older people living at home
Kelley	Michigan	117	F	47–92	Free-living	Dietary history	7	To examine relationship between nutritive quality of diets, physical well-being, and body weight
Inventory method								
Hankin	Milwaukee, Wis.	13 homes			Nursing homes	1-wk inventory (also 3-day food records for 5 individuals at each home)	5	To determine if sufficient food purchased to meet RDA and if individual meals of selected patients provided adequate nutrients

Source: P. O'Hanlon and M. B. Kohrs, "Dietary Studies of Older Americans," *The American Journal of Clinical Nutrition* 31 (July, 1978):1257–1269.

time an individual is studied. Maximum variation occurred in vitamin A intake, though its unequal distribution in foods might explain this finding.

Studies of the nutritional status of institutionalized elderly people are scarce. In one study, Justice, Howe, and Clark (1974) recorded the food intakes of elderly patients in a proprietary nursing home for five nonsuccessive days in June 1970. Some biochemical (including hematocrit and hemoglobin) and anthropometric tests (bone density) were also carried out. The most frequent diagnosis of illness among these subjects was heart or cardiovascular disease. Modified diets such as those prescribed for diabetics were included in the study.

Nutrients provided by the institutional diets equaled or exceeded the 1974 RDAs for persons in this age group. Thus cases of patient intake being insufficient to meet recommended allowances can be attributed to a failure to consume sufficient food and not to the nutrient composition of the diet. Age was not a factor in nutrient intake, though sex did exert a significant effect. Men consumed more calories than women, in addition to more carbohydrates, thiamin, and ascorbic acid. Many subjects had developed detrimental long-term food consumption habits that resulted in especially low intakes of calcium and iron. Milk, for example, was rarely consumed by half of the subjects. In addition, while no subject was served less than 5 ounces of cooked lean meat or its equivalent a day, many could or would not eat this much.

Using the guidelines applied in the Ten-State Nutrition Survey, hemoglobin values would be classified as deficient in almost all of the men and in 40 percent of the women, though pernicious anemia was not diagnosed in any of these subjects. Bone density differed significantly between men and women with approximately two-thirds of the women showing values suggesting osteoporosis. As the authors point out, however, some literature suggests that osteoporosis tends to be self-limiting with the major loss of bone occurring before 65 years of age. If this is the case, then dietary patterns before and during middle life are more significant in the development of osteoporosis than are the eating patterns of those institutionalized at an advanced age. This will be discussed in more detail in Chapter 6.

McGandy and his colleagues (1966) attempted to evaluate the relationship between age and dietary intake by controlling for socioeconomic influences. They obtained dietary records of a group of 252 apparently healthy, highly educated and successful men, most of whom were engaged in or retired from professional and managerial occupations. Subjects ranged in age from 20 to 99 and lived in the Baltimore-Washington area. Each spent two and one-half days in the hospital to participate in clinical and biochemical tests.

A marked decline in total daily calories consumed occurred with age, though RDAs for almost all nutrients, except calcium, were met by the great majority of men. In general, there was no significant decrease in nutrient intake associated with age. The authors attributed the age decrement in total daily caloric intake to decreases in basal metabolism and in energy expenditure required for physical activity. One particularly interesting finding involves a disproportionate drop in fat intake with age. This may reflect a self-imposed limitation on the part of highly educated subjects concerned about the relationship between fat intake and heart disease given so much attention by the popular media. Simple age-related changes in physiological tolerance to certain foods is another possible explanation.

Only recently have nutrition scientists begun the task of evaluating the impact of federal and state nutrition programs on the elderly. One such study, carried out by Kohrs, O'Hanlon, and Eklund (1978), reported on the contribution of a federally funded (Title VII) meal program to the total daily nutrient intake of a group of elderly people in Central Missouri. One-day food records were kept by 466 subjects—154 were participants in a meal program that day, 213 were individuals who had previously participated but did not eat the program meal that day, and 99 were nonparticipants. Those eating the meal provided by the program consumed more calories, protein, and calcium than others. Overall, they had a better quality diet than did nonparticipants, though the nonparticipants consumed more iron. Between 40 and 50 percent of total daily intake of all nutrients, except calcium, was consumed in the program meal. Women at the program meal consumed a significantly larger ratio of their intake of calories, protein, iron, and niacin than did the men. The program appears to have successfully reduced the nutritional vulnerability of its elderly participants. This reduction no doubt occurred because of the special emphasis on providing meals that contained more than one-third of the recommended daily allowances.

Data from local nutrition studies seem to corroborate data from national studies in that they broadly define the scope of nutritional vulnerability among the elderly. In addition, these local studies further emphasize the complexity of factors that may interact to affect the food intake and nutritional status of the aged. These include socioeconomic considerations such as income and education, sex, living arrangements, and the availability of meal programs to supplement dietary intake.

PROBLEMS OF DOING RESEARCH ON THE NUTRITIONAL STATUS OF THE ELDERLY

Assessing the nutritional status of a given population can be accomplished through a variety of approaches.[1] Nutrition scientists sometimes attempt an examination of a community as a whole to determine how the quality of life is related to the health and nutritional status of the group (Caliendo, 1979). This examination is often referred to as a "community assessment." According to Caliendo (1979), two basic approaches are used in a community assessment.

[1] This section relies heavily on Caliendo (1979), Evers and McIntosh (1977), and Kanawati (1976).

First, relevant vital statistics are employed to indirectly assess the community. Included here are morbidity and mortality rates, as well as other demographic and socioeconomic data. The second approach includes an assessment of cultural factors that may lead to nutritional problems. These include food consumption patterns and technological influences on food production.

More often, determination of nutritional status has been carried out by nutrition scientists through direct assessment of individuals within a community. As we have already seen from the above review of three national surveys, this face-to-face assessment can utilize four basic methods: dietary studies, anthropometry, clinical evaluation, and biochemical tests.

Dietary studies

Dietary studies are conducted to obtain accurate information on food consumption and nutrient intake. The data thus obtained is then correlated with other direct and indirect measures of nutritional status. Such studies range from food weighing and records to 24-hour recall and dietary histories. Each approach has its advantages and disadvantages.

Food records consist of recording the food consumed by an individual for a specific time, usually 3 to 7 days. A variation on food recording involves weighing actual food intake. These techniques have the advantage of providing accurate quantitative data that does not rely on subject memory. In addition, record keeping may be used over an extended period of time to help ensure that the subject's usual diet will be represented accurately. However, food recording surveys require extensive cooperation from subjects. The method of weighing food is more expensive to carry out, requires an even greater intrusion into the regular routine of participants, and is less suitable for meals not eaten in the home.

Twenty-four-hour recalls are a simple, rapid technique for obtaining information on food consumption. Generally, they can be carried out with little expense in a short period of time. A further advantage is that they can be used with a wide array of populations, though elderly people who are suffering from decrements in short-term memory can put this method to the test (Campbell and Dodds, 1967). Disadvantages include the need for a trained interviewer as well as the concern that a single 24-hour intake may not be representative of the subject's usual intake.

Diets fluctuate over time. This may be due to seasonal food availability, social change, or some unique family circumstance at a particular time (Evers and McIntosh, 1977). Thus some researchers recommend that dietary surveys be carried out at least four or five times a year in order to differentiate among seasonal, unique, and more permanent changes in a subject's situation (Exton-Smith, 1982). Dietary histories may provide an advantage in this regard over food records and estimations by recall. They generally include questions about food habits over long periods of time—sometimes as long as a full year. Thus they take into account such factors as seasonal variation in diet. On the negative side, dietary histories require trained interviewers and a high degree of cooperation from subjects. In addition, many researchers believe that the longer the duration of the study, the more that precision suffers.

Are these methods of obtaining information on dietary intake interchangeable? Several researchers have attempted to answer this question. Young and her colleagues (1952) compared the dietary history, 24-hour recall, and seven-day food record using three different population groups, none of which was elderly. The dietary history gave higher average group values for nutrient intake for two of the groups and was in better agreement with the 24-hour recall for the third group studied. However, the seven-day record and the 24-hour recall gave approximately the same estimates of dietary intake for most nutrients for all three populations. These authors suggested that under certain circumstances, the two could be interchanged in estimating group intakes.

More recently, a group of Canadian researchers (Morgan et al., 1978) compared the 24-hour recall, a detailed quantitative diet history directed to the most recent two-month period and the two-month period six months before, and a four-day diet diary on four samples of healthy subjects in Manitoba, Saskatchewan, Quebec, and Ontario. There was a relatively low correlation between the three measures, and while the authors found all methods satisfactory for determining group values, they suggest care when employing the methods to determine individual values. In particular, they note that the diet history seemed more reliable for individual estimates of usual intake. It is also preferred when current food intake may be influenced by a disease.

Gersovitz and his associates (1978) used subjects from five congregate meal sites in Blair County, Pennsylvania, to test the merits of the 24-hour dietary recall and the seven-day dietary record for group comparisons. Their data suggest that both methods provide estimates that are equally accurate relative to average intake, though subjects using the recall method appear prone to overreporting low intakes and underreporting high intakes. This tendency could be problematic in program evaluation. For instance, according to the authors, if a program such as Food Stamps does in fact improve dietary intake, the impact of such an improvement would be understated by data obtained through a method prone to overreporting low intakes and underreporting high intakes (Gersovitz et al., 1978).

Which is the best dietary survey technique? As Young and Trulson (1960) wrote over twenty years ago: "We have certainly learned that the best method to be used depends on the objective of the study and the hypothesis to be tested."

Anthropometry

Because bodily growth and development occur in recognizable patterns, any deviation can be measured and compared with normative standards for growth and development. Growth, for example, is one of the most sensitive indicators of nutritional status in children. However, we must ask if the most commonly obtained anthropometric measurements of height, weight, triceps skinfold thickness, and arm circumference (Gray and Gray, 1980) are useful for assessing the nutritional status of older adults. The answer is yes, especially when anthropometric measurements are used in conjunction with other methods.

Weight reflects current body mass but is influenced by variation in dietary intake. As a measure of malnutrition, however, weight must be evaluated in terms of actual age, height, and even in terms of what is considered a desirable weight for a given age (Bowman and Rosenberg, 1982). Height is considered to reflect long-term protein intake. Both longitudinal and cross-sectional studies indicate that height decreases with age. Rossman (1977) concludes that average life-time height loss is about 2.9 cm in men and 4.9 cm in women with approximately half the decrease in sitting height. Evers and McIntosh (1977) indicate that if only one indicator is available, height for age should be used as it reflects long-term general malnutrition. Arm circumference assesses the amount of muscle tissue and is also a measure of protein status. Triceps skinfold thickness is a measure of subcutaneous fat and can be considered an index of the body's energy stores. Interpretation of these measures is complicated by the significant changes in body composition that occur with aging, particularly reciprocal changes in lean body mass and body fat, changes in the distribution of body fat, alterations in skin thickness, turgor, elasticity, and compressibility that characterize the aging process in skin (Bowman and Rosenberg, 1982).

There are several advantages in using anthropometric measurements. One is that they are commonly in use and do not require extensive training of highly-skilled personnel. They are also relatively simple to use in the field and generally low in cost. Disadvantages include the need for precision in measurement and an accurate indication of the subject's age. Finally, anthropometry is not particularly well suited to the diagnosis of severe overt malnutrition (Robinow and Jelliffe, 1966). Even when measurements indicate the presence of nutritional deficiencies, they are not useful for detailing the nature and extent of the deficiencies—they therefore require very careful interpretation (Evers and McIntosh, 1977).

Clinical Evaluation

The clinical examination can serve as a guide for recording signs believed to be related to inadequate nutrition (Kanawati, 1976). Table 3.8 presents a list of clinical signs believed to be of value in nutrition surveys, and indicates their probable cause. As Caliendo (1979) points out, though, clinical examination of the individual is the least sensitive method that can be used to evaluate individual nutritional status. It is relatively easy to detect clinical signs of advanced overt malnutrition, but the early signs are difficult to detect and may be overlooked. Furthermore, diagnostic and interpretive capabilities vary among individuals who conduct examinations.

TABLE 3.8.   Clinical signs and their probable cause.

STRUCTURE	CLINICAL SIGNS	PROBABLE DEFICIENCY
Hair	Lack of natural shine; dull, fine, straight, stiff, color changes, brittle, wirelike.	Protein, calories
Skin	Dry, flaky, swollen, dark patches, red, black and blue marks, excessive light patches.	Protein, ascorbic acid, B vitamins
Nails	Brittle, ridged.	Protein, iron
Eyes	Dry, red, or pale membranes, redness at corners; cornea dry, soft, scarred, dull. Bitot's spots.	Vitamin A, B vitamins
Lips	Pallor of membranes, red, swollen, fissures.	Riboflavin, niacin
Tongue	Glossitis, swollen, raw, painful.	Folic acid, iron, niacin, vitamin B_{12}
	Purple tongue.	Riboflavin
Gums	Peridontal disease, spongy, receeding, bleeding, hemorrhage.	Calcium, Vitamin C
Teeth	Caries, gray or black spots, poor tooth development, mottled enamel, missing teeth.	Fluoride, vitamin D, calcium.
Glands	Enlarged thyroid.	Iodine
Extremities, bones, joints	Scrotal dermatitis.	Riboflavin
	Edema.	Protein
	Bowed legs, rachitic rosary.	Vitamin D
	Tenderness.	Thiamine
	Loss of vibration sense, tendon reflex.	Thiamine, vitamin B_{12}
	In infants, delayed closure of fontanel.	Vitamin D, calcium
	Mental irritability, burning and tingling of hands/feet, weakness.	Thiamine, vitamin B_{12}
Cardiovascular	Rapid heart rate, enlarged heart, abnormal rhythm.	Protein, minerals chronic malnutrition
Gastrointestinal	Enlarged liver, spleen.	Chronic malnutrition

Source: Mary Alice Caliendo, *Nutrition and the World Food Crisis*. New York, Macmillan, 1979. Reprinted with permission of Macmillan Publishing Co., Inc. © 1979 by Mary Alice Caliendo.

Biochemical tests

Biochemical tests are used to determine the body's stores of particular nutrients and to evaluate certain functions which are dependent on the supply of particular nutrients. These tests are particularly useful because nutrient stores may become depleted long before clinical and anthropometric changes are evident. Table 3.9 gives a list of laboratory tests for nutrients and metabolites. These tests are classified into "first category" and "second category" according to their practicality in the field. The precision and accuracy of the results of such tests vary according to the particular nutrient tested for and the conditions under which the tests are carried out and analyzed (Evers and McIntosh, 1977). While the tests are highly reliable, some controversy exists over what the cutoff point should be when determining "normal" and deficient values (Thurnham, 1975).

Nutritional status is complex. It is affected by a multiplicity of factors, including socioeconomic and cultural complications, which makes its measurement difficult. Compounding these factors are, as we have already suggested, problems of precision, reliability, and validity that plague all the existing devices used for measurement. One research strategy that overcomes

TABLE 3.9.   Laboratory tests for nutrients and metabolites.

NUTRIENT	1ST CATEGORY	2ND CATEGORY
Protein	Plasma amino acids, urinary hydroxyproline, serum albumin urinary urea/creatinine	Total serum protein
Lipids	Serum cholesterol, triglycerides, lipoproteins	
Vitamin A	Serum vitamin A and carotene	
Vitamin D	Serum 250H cholecalciferol serum alkaline phosphatase	Serum calcium and phosphorous
Ascorbic acid	Whole blood ascorbic acid	
Thiamine	Urinary thiamine, erythrocyte transketolase activity	Blood pyruvate
Riboflavin	Urinary riboflavin, erythrocyte glutathione reductase	
Nicotinic acid		N_1-Methyl nicotinamide and its ⁶pyridone in urine
Folic acid	Red cell folate	Serum folate, bone marrow film, thin blood film
Vitamin B_{12}	Serum vitamin B_{12}, serum thymidylate synthetase, urine methylmalonic acid	Bone marrow film Thin blood film Schilling test
Iron	Iron deposits in bone marrow, serum iron and % saturation of transferrin	Haemoglobin Haematocrit Thin blood film
Iodine		Urinary iodine Tests for thyroid function

Source: Abdallah Kanawati, "Assessment of Nutritional Status in the Community," in D. McLaren (ed.), *Nutrition in the Community*. London, John Wiley & Sons, 1976.

the weaknesses of several measurement devices is called *triangulation* and involves the use of multiple measurement techniques (Williamson, Karp and Dalphin, 1977). Since the function of triangulation is to affirm the validity of measures, what is required are measures that are independent of one another and based on different types of data. The methods of nutritional assessment discussed above—dietary studies, anthropometry, clinical examination, and biochemical testing—meet the criterion of independence and thus can be used for purposes of triangulation. Until now, nutrition researchers using a triangulated package of methods have employed all four measurement approaches. This was the case in the Ten-State Survey and the HANES primarily because the best combination of methods has yet to be determined.

FUTURE RESEARCH NEEDS

In many respects, data on the nutritional status of older Americans are quite sparse. Clearly, more research at the national level is necessary. The Ten-State Survey and the HANES are more than ten years old, and these studies were not specific to the elderly. The aged are a heterogeneous group. Emphasis must be placed on quantifying the nutritional status of important subgroups of this population, which include the poor, those with disease, the institutionalized, the healthy, and the nonwhite aged. While in recent years we have become enlightened about the impact of income and health status on the nutritional position of the elderly, it is important to further tease out the additional socio-economic and cultural determinants of nutrient intake and nutritional status.

Development of more valid and reliable measures of nutritional status is essential. In addition, systematic research on triangulated methods of assessment would advance the state of the art immeasurably. Indirect methods of assessing the nutritional status of the elderly also need further evaluation.

In the last decade or so, several important public and private programs have been initiated in order to favorably affect the nutritional status of elderly Americans. These programs are grand experiments in nutritional intervention. Though we will not discuss these programs until later in this book (Chapter 7), it seems appropriate at this point to suggest the need for evaluation of these intervention strategies.

SUMMARY

National surveys, including the Department of Agriculture's Household Food Consumption Survey, the Ten-State Survey, and the HANES, seem to indicate that large numbers of the elderly population are nutritionally vulnerable. Those with low income and the sick and disabled are particularly susceptible. In fact, the nutritional status of the elderly seems more tied to income and health status than to age per se.

Local and regional studies lend support to the picture drawn from the national data. In addition, these studies further emphasize the complexity of factors that interact to affect nutrient intake and the nutritional status of the aged. These factors include education, sex, and living arrangements.

Researchers use indirect and direct methods of assessing nutritional status. The former, including morbidity and mortality rates, are often employed in a "community assessment." The latter involve face-to-face assessment of individuals in the community and include dietary studies, anthropometry, clinical evaluation, and biochemical testing. Problems of precision, reliability and validity plague all the above existing measurement devices. Because of these problems, triangulation, which involves using multiple measurement techniques, seems a fruitful strategy to employ in nutrition research.

STUDY QUESTIONS

1. What do the national surveys tell us about caloric and nutrient intake among the elderly? How do the elderly compare with younger population groups represented in the national studies?
2. What is the relationship between income and nutritional status among the elderly? Use the data from the three national surveys cited in the text to support your view.
3. Local nutrition studies seem to emphasize the complexity of factors that may interact to affect the food intake and nutritional status of the aged. Use those studies cited in the text to describe how nutrient and caloric intake may vary according to education, sex, and the living arrangements of the elderly.
4. Why do researchers carry out dietary studies? Identify two methods of dietary study and indicate the special advantages and disadvantages of each.
5. Are anthropometric measurements useful for assessing the nutritional status of older people? What are the advantages and disadvantages of these techniques?
6. Compare and contrast clinical evaluation and biochemical testing as techniques for evaluating nutritional status. What are the respective problems of precision, reliability, and validity that plague these techniques?
7. Define triangulation. How is it useful to nutrition scientists?
8. Where would you place the emphasis for future research on the nutritional status of the aged?

BIBLIOGRAPHY

BARROWS, C. H. and ROEDER, L. M., "Nutrition," in C. E. Finch and L. Hayflick (eds.), *Handbook of the Biology of Aging.* New York, Van Nostrand Reinhold, 1977.

BOWMAN, B. B. and ROSENBERG, I. H., "Assessment of the Nutritional Status of the Elderly," *American Journal of Clinical Nutrition,* 35 (1982), 1142–1151.

CALIENDO, M. A., *Nutrition and the World Food Crisis.* New York, Macmillan, 1979.

CAMPBELL, V. A. and DODDS, M. L., Collecting Dietary Information from Groups of Older People," *Journal of American Dietetic Assn.,* 51(1967), 29–33.

CLARKE, M. and WAKEFIELD, L., "Food Choices of Institutionalized vs. Independent-living Elderly," *Journal American Dietetic Assn.,* 66(1975), 600–604.

DAVIDSON, C. S., LIVERMORE, J., ANDERSON, P., and KAUFMAN, S., "The Nutrition of a Group of Apparently Healthy Aging Persons," *American Journal of Clinical Nutrition,* 10(1962), 181

DIBBLE, M. V., BRIN, M., THIELE, V. F., PEEL, A., CHEN, N., and MCMULLEN, C., "Evaluation of the Nutritional Status of Elderly Subjects with a Comparison Between Fall and Spring," *Journal American Geriatrics Society,* 15(1967), 1031–1061.

EVERS, S. and MCINTOSH, W. A., "Social Indicators of Human Nutrition," *Social Indicators Research,* 4(1977), 185–205.

EXTON-SMITH, A. N., "Epidemiological Studies in the Elderly: Methodological Considerations," *American Journal of Clinical Nutrition,* 35(1982), 1273–1279.

FRY, P., FOX, H., and LINKSWILER, H., "Nutrient Intakes of Healthy Older Women," *Journal American Dietetic Assn.,* 42(1963), 218–222.

GERSOVITZ, M., MADDEN, J. P., and SMICIKLAS-WRIGHT, H., "Validity of the 24-hour Dietary Recall and Seven-day Record for Group Comparisons," *Journal of American Dietetic Assn.,* 73(1978), 48–55.

GOODMAN, S., *Assessment of Nutritional Impact of Congregate Meals Program for the Elderly.* Unpublished Ph.D. Thesis, Pennsylvania State Univ., 1974.

GRAY, G. E. and GRAY, L. K., "Anthropometric Mesurements and Their Interpretation," *Journal of American Dietetic Assn.,* 77(1980), 534–539.

GREGER, J. and SCISCOE, B., "Zinc Nutriture of Elderly Participants in an Urban Feeding Program," *Journal American Dietetic Assn.,* 70(1977), 37–41.

GUTHRIE, H., BLACK, K., and MADDEN, J., "Nutritional Practices of Elderly Citizens in Rural Pennsylvania," *Gerontologist,* 12(1972), 330–335.

HANKIN, J. and ANTONMATTEI, J., "Survey of Food Practices in Nursing Homes," *American Journal Public Health,* 59(1960), 1137–1144.

HARRILL, I., ERBES, C., and SCHWARTZ, C., "Observations on Food Acceptance by Elderly Women," *Gerontologist,* 16(1976), 349–355.

JOERING, E., "Nutrient Contribution of a Meals Program for Senior Citizens," *Journal American Dietetic Assn.,* 59(1971), 129–132.

JUSTICE, C., HOWE, J., and CLARK, H., "Dietary Intakes and Nutritional Status of Elderly Patients," *Journal American Dietetic Assn.,* 65(1974), 639–646.

KANAWATI, A., "Assessment of Nutritional Status in the Community," in D. McLaren (ed.), *Nutrition in the Community.* London, John Wiley, 1976.

KELLEY, L., OHLSON, M., and HARPER, L., "Food Selection and Well-Being of Aging Women," *Journal of American Dietetic Assn.,* 33(1957), 466–470.

KOHRS, M., O'HANLON, P., and EKLUND, D., "Contribution of the Older American's Nutrition Programs to One Day's Dietary Intake," *Journal American Dietetic Assn.,* 72(1978), 487–492.

KOHRS, M. B.,   et al., "Nutritional Status of Elderly Residents in Missouri," *American Journal of Clinical Nutrition*, 31 (1978), 2186–2197.

LEBOVIT, C., "The Food Of Older Persons Living at Home," *Journal American Dietetic Assn.*, 46(1965), 285–289.

LYONS, J. C. and TRULSON, M. F., "Food Practices of Older People Living at Home," *Journal Gerontology*, 11(1956), 66

MCGANDY, R. B., BARROWS, C. H., SPANIAS, G., MEREDITH, A., STONE, J. L., and NORRIS, A. H., "Nutrient Intakes and Energy Expenditures in Men of Different Ages," *Journal Gerontology*, 21(1966), 581–587.

MORGAN, R. W., JAIN, M., MILLER, A. B., CHOI, N. W., MATHEWS, V., MUNAN, L., BURTH, J. D., FEATHER, J., HOWE, G. R., and KELLY, A., "A Comparison of Dietary Methods in Epidemiologic Studies," *American Journal of Epidemiology*, 107(1978), 488–498.

National Center for Health Statistics, *First Health and Nutrition Example Survey, U. S., 1971–1972*. DHEW Publ. No. (HRA) 74-1219-1 Health Services Admin. Washington, D. C., Government Printing Office, 1974.

Nutrition Canada, *National Survey, 1970–72*. Ottawa, Information Canada, 1973.

O'HANLON, P. and KOHRS, M. B., "Dietary Studies of Older Americans," *American Journal of Clinical Nutrition*, 31(1978), 1257–1269.

OHLSON, M. A., JACKSON, A. L., BOEK, J., CEDERQUIST, D. D., BREWER, W. D., and BROWN, E. G., "Nutrition and Dietary Habits of Aging Women," *American Journal of Public Health*, 49(1950), 1101–1108.

ROBINOW, M. and JELIFFE, D. B., "Intercorrelations Between Anthropometric Variables," *Proceedings of the Seventh Int'l Congress of Nutrition*, 4(1966), 140–145.

ROSSMAN, I., "Anatomic and Body Composition Changes with Aging," in C. E. Finch and L. Hayflick (eds.), *op. cit.*, 189–221.

STEINKAMP, R., COHEN, N., and WALSH, J., "Re-Survey of an Aging Population—14 Years Follow-up," *Journal American Dietetic Assn.*, 46(1965), 103–110.

THURNHAM, D. L., "The Range and Variability of Biochemical Indices: What is 'Normal'?" *Nutrition*, 29(1975), 79.

TODHUNTER, E., HOUSE, F., and VANDER ZWAGG, R., *Food Acceptance and Food Attitudes of the Elderly*. Nashville, Tennessee Commission on Aging, 1974.

TUCKER, R., BRINE, C., and WALLACE, M., "Nutritive Intake of Older Institutionalized Persons," *Journal American Dietetic Assn.*, 34(1958), 819–822.

U. S. Department of Agriculture, *Consumption of Households in the U. S., Spring, 1965*. Dept. No. 1. Washington, D. C., Government Printing Office, 1968.

U. S. Department of Health, Education, and Welfare, *Ten-State Nutrition Survey, 1968-1970. Anthropometric and Clinical Findings*. DHEW Publ. No. (HRA) 75-1229 Health Resources Administration. Washington, D. C., Government Printing Office, 1975.

WATKIN, D., "Nutritional Problems Today in the Elderly in the U. S.," in A. Exton-Smith and D. Scott (eds.), *Vitamins in the Elderly*. Bristol, England, John Wright and Sons, 1968.

WILLIAMSON, J. B., KARP, D. A., and DALPHIN, J. R., *The Research Craft*. Boston, Little, Brown, 1977.

YOUNG, C. M., HAGAN, G. C., TUCKER, R. E., and FOSTER, W. D., "A Comparison of Dietary Study Methods," *Journal of American Dietetic Assn.*, 28(1952), 218–221.

YOUNG, C. M. and TRULSON, M. F., "Methodology for Dietary Studies in Epidemiological Surveys, II," *American Journal of Public Health*, 50(1960), 803–814.

CHAPTER FOUR
NUTRITIONAL
NEEDS IN OLD AGE

Nutrients are chemical constituents of food necessary for proper body functioning. They supply us with energy, aid in the growth and repair of body tissues, and are involved in the regulation of body processes. Some nutrients perform all three functions.

Presently, there are six major accepted categories of nutrients: carbohydrates, fat, protein, vitamins, minerals and water. Although all types of dietary fiber (except lignin) are recognized as carbohydrates, fiber is not yet recognized as an essential nutrient. However, fiber should not be ignored in a consideration of the food constituents essential to proper body functioning. This nondigestible portion of plant food adds bulk to the diet and is important in maintaining intestinal motility. Some epidemiologic data indicate that it may be an important variable in the prevention of such disorders as colon cancer and cardiovascular disease. The role of dietary fiber in disease processes will be discussed in greater detail in Chapter 6.

Although the categories of nutrients are well recognized, the specific amounts of each nutrient needed for optimal functioning is a matter of much controversy. Scientists debate among themselves about how much of a particular nutrient is needed on a daily basis to assure the body's efficient performance. Some nutritionists seem to vie for public recognition of their theories regarding what constitutes sound dietary practice. Perhaps part of the reason for confusion in this area is the fact that the field of nutritional science is relatively young. It was not until the founding of the American Institute of Nutrition in 1934 that nutrition became officially identified as a separate discipline of study. Atwater, Rose, Lusk, McCallum, and others pioneered the study of nutritional science, especially in the area of energy balance and vitamin deficiency. Since then, much more has been learned about animal nutrition than human nutrition as research priorities have centered around such issues as the cost-benefit concerns of raising livestock for a profit. However, our knowledge is increasing and hopefully will continue to do so as more research on human nutrition is undertaken.

DIETARY STANDARDS

Two kinds of "standards" are involved in a consideration of the nutritional requirements of the elderly (and everyone else, for that matter). Intake at levels of *minimal requirements* of certain nutrients prevent the development of overt symptoms of nutritional deficiency disease. *Optimal requirement* intake provides nutrients at levels that should assure the maintenance of optimal health in most individuals. For the most part, nutritional scientists agree upon the minimal requirements, but the optimal requirements sometimes are subject to controversy. Much of this controversy surrounds the concept of *Recommended Dietary Allowances* (RDAs), which originated as a result of human population surveys used to determine health status in relation to nutrient intake, controlled human feeding experiments, and animal studies on metabolism. The RDAs, as shown in Table 4.1, do not represent minimal or optimal requirements. They are intended as reference points for planning diets for all groups of people to provide the greatest health benefits. The RDAs are continually being researched, and revisions are made approximately every five years.

Previously, it was believed that the nutritional requirements of the elderly were quite similar to those of other age groups. New data have contributed to a change in this belief. For example, it is now clear that the progressive physical changes associated with aging are capable of affecting nutritional requirements. Changes in digestive functions, enzyme producing organs, intestinal mucosa, and kidney functioning influence the speed and efficiency with which food is digested, nutrients are absorbed, and the residual matter excreted (Brocklehurst, 1979). Age-related changes in blood vessels influence their ability to nourish body tissues at the levels they once did. Disease associated with age may also directly or indirectly modify nutrient needs. More research is needed in this area to provide a better understanding of how the progress of different diseases interacts with age-related changes to modify nutrient needs. It is already known that in many instances drugs used to treat disease can also affect nutritional status. However, all of these factors exhibit a great deal of variability in their manifestations in particular aged individuals.

TABLE 4.1   Recommended Dietary Allowances (RDAs) 1980, for individuals 51 to 75 years of age.

	MALES	FEMALES
Fat Soluble Vitamins		
A	1,000 μg. R.E.[1]	800 μg. R.E.[1]
D Cholecalciferal	5 μg.	5 μg.
E	10 T.E.[2]	8 T.E.[2]
K	70–140 μg.	70–140 μg.
Water Soluble Vitamins		
C	60 mg.	60 mg.
Thiamin	1.2 mg.	1.0 mg.
Riboflavin	1.4 mg.	1.2 mg.
Niacin	16 mg.	13 mg.
B_6	2.2 mg.	2.0 mg.
Folic Acid	400 μg.	400 μg.
B_{12}	3.0 μg.	3.0 μg.
Pantothenic Acid	4–7 mg.	4–7 mg.
Biotin	100–200 μg.	100–200 μg.
Energy		
Age 51-75	2400[3] calories	1800[4] calories
Over 75	2050[3] calories	1600[4] calories
Protein		
	56 grams	44 grams

[1]R.E. = Retinol Equivalents
[2]T.E. = Tocopherol Equivalents
[3]For men average height 70 inches, 154 pounds
[4]For women average height 64 inches, 120 pounds
Source: National Research Council, Food and Nutrition Board, 1980. *Recommended Dietary Allowances, Revised 1980.* (Washington, D.C.: National Research Council - National Academy of Sciences).

Social factors associated with aging may also affect the nutritional requirements of older people. For example, older persons may be more vulnerable to protein deficiency as sociocultural and physical stresses contribute to the excretion of nitrogen, an important constituent of protein. This deficiency may be exacerbated by low consumption of protein and the presence of absorption problems.

As we have already seen, the problem of assessing nutritional adequacy in the elderly is not a simple one. Yet it is an essential stage in formulating sound ideas on the possibility of variable nutritional needs of the elderly. The major assessment problems for clinicians, planners, and researchers may be characterized as follows:

1) Many of the changes associated with the aging process often overlap or imitate the signs of a nutritional deficiency. For example, vascular "spiders" under the tongue are often noted as a sign of vitamin C deficiency. In most cases, they are simply a sign of increased capillary fragility associated with aging.

2) Some nutrient deficiencies have nonspecific symptoms, and some of these symptoms may be due to deficiency of one or more of several nutrients.

3) Chronic disease or other disorders may alter the nutritional requirements for an affected individual.

4) Diseases with a related nutritional component (such as osteoporosis or periodontal disease) may be associated with a poor dietary history. What we eat throughout life influences our nutritional status in later years.

5) Little is known about "biochemical individuality" and nutritional needs.

6) The use of vitamin supplements is believed to be widespread among the elderly. Such usage might not be accounted for in surveys of dietary adequacy. It is possible for vitamin supplementation to upset dynamic balances among nutrients, thus altering the "normal" requirements of a given nutrient or nutrients.

7) The impact of age is variable among individuals—each individual is a unique sum of life experiences, diseases, and the aging process. However, most changes are more marked and possibly more uniform after age 75. However, the aged are far more heterogeneous as a group than are other population groups.

Keeping these problems in mind, let us briefly survey the major nutrient categories and their relationship to aging individuals.

CALORIES

Most nutritionists agree that there is a strong case for recommending a reduced intake of calories for the elderly. Calories represent measures of food energy and are derived from three nutrients: carbohydrates, fats, and protein. In general, the energy needs of the elderly decline due to a reduction of activity and a slowing of the basal metabolism rate (BMR), although the former may fall the more drastically of the two. The BMR refers to the amount of energy which the lean body mass needs in order to carry out its basic functions. With age, there is a decline in the ratio of lean body mass to fat, which results in a lower BMR since the metabolic needs of fat tissue are less than those of lean. Even for those who exercise regularly, there is a decrease in the number of calories that need to be consumed.

According to the National Research Council (1980), the rate of reduction of caloric needs is individually variable but may approximate five percent per decade between ages 55 and 75, and seven percent per decade after the age of 75. The amount of reduced energy needs also varies with an individual's size and level of physical activity. Disease and disability complicate the situation in two ways. They can contribute to inactivity and decreased energy needs or lead to increased energy demands for the performance of certain tasks due to various kinds of increased stress and strain.

Reduced activity itself may be related to motivational state, retirement, or chronic disease. Activity is valuable for the health and well being of the elderly individual for a variety of reasons, including the following:

1) It requires energy expenditure, thus helping to maintain an energy balance and aiding in the avoidance of obesity.
2) It leads to greater activity and increases work capacity, both of which lead to greater consumption of calories. Failure to consume adequate calories can contribute to fatigue and lassitude.
3) It prevents or slows atrophy associated with chronic disease and inactivity by maintaining good muscle tone.
4) It lowers blood sugar levels, often improving glucose tolerance and lowering insulin dosage level in diabetics.
5) It is stimulating and may serve to lift an individual's spirits.

Although caloric needs are reduced in later life, the need for specific nutrients does not decrease. Quantitative and qualitative variety must be included in the diet in order to provide the necessary amounts of all essential nutrients. However, it must be emphasized that adequate calorie consumption is necessary to allow for a sufficient intake of the essential nutrients.

CARBOHYDRATE NEEDS

Carbohydrates constitute a major portion of most diets including those of the elderly. Over the years, they have developed an undeserved reputation as the cause of weight gain. Certainly this energy-yielding nutrient can contribute to excess weight if it is part of an overall dietary plan that includes too many calories. For instance, many of the so-called snack and junk foods are high in calories, refined carbohydrates, and fats, and low in other nutrients. However, cookies, crackers, pastries, and doughnuts are not the only foods in the carbohydrate category. It is also represented by the complex carbohydrates found in fruits, vegetables, cereals, and breads. These foods are also rich in protective nutrients such as vitamins and minerals. Carbohydrates are the main sources of dietary fiber. It is recommended that the majority of calories consumed consist of complex carbohydrates in the form of the above-mentioned foods. Foods high in refined sugars, though a source of pleasure to many, should be eaten in moderation. This avoids unnecessary increments in energy intake. Such advice regarding carbohydrated consumption applies to persons in all age categories.

PROTEIN NEEDS

It appears that protein needs are similar in both the young and the old. However, there are important physical and social factors to consider in the case of the older adult that may increase the likelihood of a marginal protein status. Poor chewing ability and the expense of protein-rich foods can limit protein intake. Substituting dairy products or eggs for harder to chew meats may pose other difficulties. They are expensive, and milk may not be tolerated due to a lactase deficiency or merely because the adult has not regularly included it in the diet since youth. Transporting heavy cartons of milk may also be no easy task, especially for the socially isolated individual who has no one to aid him or her in shopping.

In addition to the above-mentioned problems, some adults may be advised by a physician to curtail intake of red meat and unskimmed dairy products because of the high cholesterol and saturated fat content of these foods. Fish, poultry, and combinations of plant foods can supply the necessary protein in the diet. Animal products are known as complete proteins which means that they supply all of the eight essential amino acids, or building-blocks, for protein. In general, plant foods contain smaller amounts of protein than animal products and, in most cases, are lower in one or more of the essential amino acids. Proteins that do not have the proper balance of essential amino acids are known as incomplete proteins. One can achieve a better protein balance by combining plant foods. For example, casseroles containing beans and rice are complete in their amino acid content and are an easy-to-chew, less expensive, "steak substitute."

It has been noted that increased stress leads to higher rates of nitrogen excretion, which may result in a negative nitrogen balance (Young, 1976, 1978). Since the elderly are potentially subject to multiple stress factors, including role changes, increased risk of illness, and multiple disease states, "normal" protein intake may be insufficient for optimal health. Decreased ability to absorb nutrients, related to age-induced changes in the digestive system, affects protein balance. Evidence is presently inconclusive in support of the contention that the elderly have increased needs for the amino acids lysine and methionine (Young, 1976).

It has also been suggested that protein needs may be reduced in old age. Such suggestions are related to the observations that body protein mass declines with age (Forbes and Reina, 1970) and that the rate of protein synthesis decreases (Winterer et al., 1976). Declining renal function may also make it difficult to handle high concentrations of protein waste (this is discussed in Chapter 6).

FAT NEEDS

Age does not alter an individual's need for fat. Fats should be limited to less than 25–30 percent of total caloric intake at all ages. Reducing fat consumption is an easy way to reduce the total intake of calories. Although the data are conflicting, the relation of fat consumption to cardiovascular disease (discussed in Chapter 6) must be considered in dietary planning even though there is no *conclusive* evidence to indicate that modifying fat intake in older persons will influence the risk of heart attack or stroke.

Restricting fat intake too drastically may interfere with absorption of fat-soluble vitamins. Besides serving as a carrier of certain vitamins and an essential fatty acid, linolec acid, fats are important in the diet for flavor and satiety. A totally fat-free diet would be monotonous, tasteless and counterproductive to good eating habits. Furthermore, we must consider that fat absorption often decreases as one ages, and that consequently absorption time is lengthened. This situation is related to several factors including a decreased production of pancreatic lipase (a fat splitting enzyme), gall bladder and liver disorders that decrease fat emulsification, and structural changes in the intestinal mucosa that interfere with fat absorption.

VITAMIN NEEDS

Vitamins are receiving greater attention these days by nutrition-conscious people of all ages. Table 4.2 describes the many dietary sources of essential vitamins. Many people, unsure of the state of their vitamin intake, seek insurance, or "super-effects," by turning to the use of vitamin supplements. The elderly are no exception to this practice. Although there is some evidence of vitamin deficiencies among the aged (See Chapter 3), there seems to be little justification for wholesale vitamin supplementation of older people. However, it might be useful to selectively supplement "at risk" groups such as elderly men living alone, those with physical disorders or sensory impairment, the re-

TABLE 4.2 Major dietary sources of essential vitamins.

Fat-Soluble Vitamins
A —milk, butter, cheese, liver, and fortified margarine (retinol)
 —green and yellow vegetables and fruits (carotene)
D —cod liver oil, fortified milk and margarine, liver, fatty fish, eggs
E —seeds, nuts, green leafy vegetables, corn oil margarines, oils such as corn, safflower
K —green leafy vegetables, liver

Water-Soluble Vitamins

Thiamin	—pork, organ meats, whole grains, legumes
Riboflavin	—milk, eggs, cheese, meats, green vegetables, legumes
Niacin	—liver, lean meats, whole grains, legumes
B_6	—whole grains, meat, vegetables, bananas, legumes
Pantothenic Acid	—organ meats, eggs, legumes, whole grains
Folacin	—legumes, whole wheat, green vegetables
B_{12}*	—organ meats, muscle meats, eggs, shellfish, liver, dairy products
C	—citrus fruit, tomatoes, green peppers, cabbage, potatoes, other fruit (melon, strawberries) other dark green leafy vegetables

*No known plant source

cently bereaved, and those suffering from depression.

Vitamin supplementation is not without problems. Vitamin absorption or storage may be affected by organs that are no longer functioning optimally due to age-related changes in organ structure and function. A field study by Baker and his colleagues (1980) demonstrated that because of vitamin malabsorption in the elderly, intramuscular vitamin injections may be necessary to maintain adequate blood levels of certain vitamins. A few vitamins pose the threat of toxic effects in those engaged in overzealous consumption. Furthermore, vitamin supplementation can disturb the dynamic interrelationships among certain nutrients. With these points in mind, let us examine specific vitamin needs during the later years.

Fat-Soluble Vitamins

The fat-soluble vitamins are A, D, E, and K. These vitamins are absorbed in the small intestine and carried by digested dietary fats. The body stores these vitamins mostly in the liver. Toxic symptoms can result from the storage of excess levels of vitamins A and D.

Vitamin A promotes healthy epithelial tissues, tooth growth and tooth enamel development in children, and the ability to see in dim light. It has also been shown to have a role in carbohydrate metabolism and may serve in an anti-infective capacity through its role in normal mucus formation. Healthy mucous membranes that are bathed in their secretions provide a more effective barrier to the invasion of various pathogenic micro-organisms. Some investigators have also reported a correlation between a low intake of vitamin A and a susceptibility to chemical carcinogens affecting the respiratory system, colon, and urinary bladder (Wald, 1980).

Vitamin A deficiencies can result from poor intake, poor intestinal absorption, or from diseases that affect the utilization of vitamin A. In the elderly, vitamin A deficiency is most likely to become a problem due to impaired absorption or disease rather than because of underconsumption. A variety of factors can lead to poor absorption. These include a reduced availability of bile (important in the emulsification of fats), overuse of laxatives, antibiotic therapy, and cirrhosis of the liver. Increasing dysfunction of the gall bladder and liver are often associated with aging and can lead to unavailability of bile due to physical obstruction as well as its inadequate production by the liver. Low levels of bile disrupt fat digestion and absorption as well as absorption of the fat-soluble vitamins. Laxative use, which is high in the elderly, may serve to flush this vitamin out of the body. Oil-based laxatives (such as mineral oil) act as carriers of vitamin A and are especially significant in the disruption of absorption of vitamin A.

Antibiotic therapy may introduce disruptive ecological changes in the digestive tract and can result in altered absorption of nutrients. Cirrhosis of the liver, common in elderly alcoholics, affects the ability of the liver to metabolize and store vitamin A.

The primary function of vitamin D appears to be in the area of aiding in the absorption of calcium for maintenance of healthy bone tissue. It contributes to this function by increasing the absorption of calcium from the small intestine and increasing the rate of bone mineralization. Common factors associated with a deficiency of this nutrient in the elderly are malabsorption syndromes and limited exposure to the sun. Sunlight converts a biologically inactive substance in the skin, 7-dehydrocholesterol, to vitamin D. Available information on vitamin D metabolism and the elderly is limited. Osteomalacia (see Chapter 6), the adult counterpart of rickets, has been observed in the elderly living alone. This condition is probably the result of a complex set of factors including reduced outdoor activity (which reduces exposure to sunlight), malabsorption, declining renal function (which influences calcium resorption), as well as inadequate intake of vitamin D. A deficiency of vitamin D and calcium can be most severe in its effects on skeletal integrity.

Vitamin E has been championed by faddists as a panacea for a variety of ailments and conditions (Roberts,1981). It is claimed to be a relevant factor in improving conditions ranging from heart disease to a poor-quality sex life. A great number of its alleged benefits appeal to the elderly. In fact, the antioxidant qualities of the vitamin are presumed by some to fight or retard the aging process itself (Roberts, 1981). Few of vitamin E's suggested benefits have been confirmed by well controlled scientific research, although some evidence suggest a higher requirement for older populations (Machlin and Brin, 1980).

Vitamin E is necessary for the integrity of the red blood cell and for the proper metabolism of polyunsaturated fats. Its supplementation has improved a painful leg condition known as claudication. Deficiency of vitamin E has rarely been observed except in premature infants and has proven exceptionally hard to induce in control populations (Horwitt, 1976).

Vitamin K is essential for the formation of prothrombin in the liver and thus is necessary for proper blood clotting. Deficiency of this vitamin has never been reported in healthy adults. However, low levels of vitamin K may be related to bleeding tendencies often associated with biliary disease and surgery. Likewise, availability of this vitamin may be affected by antibiotic therapy that disrupts the vitamin K producing flora of the intestine and by disease such as colitis that affect the absorptive mucosa of the small intestine.

Vitamin K deficiency is not a major problem among the elderly. However, blood levels of this vitamin should be checked and possibly supplemented because of its importance in proper blood clotting when preparing elderly persons for surgery.

Water-Soluble Vitamins

The water-soluble vitamins include the B-complex vitamins and vitamin C. Sometimes termed labile, water-soluble vitamins taken in excess of daily needs are excreted in the urine. They differ from the fat-soluble vitamins in that they normally do not accumulate in toxic quantities, though symptomatic changes have been observed in those taking megadoses of some B vitamins. It is possible, however, that excessive amounts of water-soluble vitamins may alter the dynamic balance among other nutrients or increase the need for some others. More studies are needed to determine the risk of kidney damage as a result of ingesting consistent excesses of the water-soluble vitamins. Many of these vitamins are subject to destruction as a result of food preparation and cooking practices, especially when large amounts of water are involved.

B-complex vitamins include thiamin (B_1), riboflavin (B_2), niacin, vitamin B_6 (pyridoxine), folacin (folic acid), vitamin B_{12}, biotin, and pantothenic acid. These vitamins differ chemically, but their functions are interrelated.

Thiamin has an important role in the process that changes glucose to energy. It functions as part of a coenzyme that is indispensable in carbohydrate metabolism, providing a supply of energy to the nerves and brain. Because of this relationship, thiamin deficiency usually involves neurological manifestations and mood changes. Thiamin also appears to be essential for fat and protein metabolism. Poorly balanced or highly refined diets, stress, alcoholism, and impaired intestinal absorption are most often the precipitating factors in thiamin deficiency.

Serum levels of thiamin are often reported to be low in surveys of older populations. Frequent use of diuretics can contribute to a deficiency as a result of increased excretion. The high carbohydrate diets often consumed by the elderly on marginal or fixed incomes can disturb the thiamin-carbohydrate balance, leading to a deficiency because of thiamin's role in the proper utilization of carbohydrates (Wilson, 1975; Brin and Bauernfeind, 1978). Compared to the young, the elderly may need more thiamin because of age-associated health conditions. Common among these conditions are elevated temperature, malignancy, parenteral administration of glucose without thiamin, hemodialysis (which removes thiamin), the stress of surgery, and alcoholism.

Whanger (1973) has suggested that thiamin may be inactivated in older people due to a lack of hydrochloric acid in gastric secretions and altered intestinal flora that binds ingested thiamin. Cheraskin and his colleagues (1967) suggested a relationship between low thiamin intake and greater frequency of cardiovascular complaints in older people. Thiamin intake and status should be regularly monitored in the elderly.

Riboflavin is essential for normal tissue maintenance, tear production, and corneal integrity. It is also a constituent of enzymes important in energy metabolism. Deficiencies are often associated with high carbohydrate diets lacking in animal protein, milk, and vegetables. Visual impairments, such as sensitivity to bright light, and skin problems such as epithelial lesions are common signs of a deficiency. Deficiencies of riboflavin have been reported with some regularity in the elderly. Some have suggested that it might be the most common subclinical deficiency among the elderly poor whose diets are notoriously low in meats and vegetables (for example, see Exton-Smith, 1968, 1978).

Niacin is a functional component of coenzymes that are essential for the release of energy from carbohydrates, fats, and proteins. It also plays a significant role in the synthesis of fats and protein by the body. Niacin can be *endogenously* manufactured rather inefficiently from the amino acid tryptophan (60 mg. of tryptophan yields 1 mg. of niacin). Niacin deficiency is associated with narrow, maize-dominated diets or highly refined diets limited in animal protein. Alcoholics, food faddists, and those with malabsorption problems may also suffer from niacin deficiency.

Niacin deficiency is rarely reported among the elderly, with the exception of elderly alcoholics. Those on heavy aspirin therapy for conditions such as arthritis are at risk since aspirin may interfere with the passage of niacin from plasma to tissue. Some personality changes observed in the elderly and usually attributed to the aging process, such as mental confusion and depression, may be due to deficiency of niacin as well as other B-complex deficiencies (Exton-Smith, 1968, 1978).

The vitamin B_6 group includes three closely related components that serve as coenzymes for biological functions involving amino acid metabolism and protein synthesis. It seems to be poorly absorbed by those with liver disease and is commonly deficient in persons with uremia and gastrointestinal disease. Since these conditions are often present in the elderly, these relationships bear watching.

The drug dihydroxyphenylalanine (L-dopa), a neurotransmitter, is used in treatment of Parkinson's disease. The B_6 vitamin, pyridoxin, enhances the conversion of L-dopa to dopamine. Since dopamine cannot cross the blood brain barrier, such conversion may result in a nullification of the therapeutic effects of the drug. Therefore persons on L-dopa drug therapy should avoid taking vitamin supplements containing vitamin B_6.

Folic acid (or folacin) is important in the metabolism of a number of amino and nucleic acids, and especially in hemoglobin synthesis. This vitamin's activities are interrelated with those of vitamin B_{12}. Folacin intake is frequently reported as low among the elderly. It may be the most common deficiency in the older adult (Girdwood et al., 1967), while Herbert (1967) suggests that it is the most common overall nutritional deficiency. A number of conditions often associated with old age affect folic acid availability. Surgery of the stomach and small intestine are associated with decreased absorption of the vitamin. Leukemia, Hodgkin's disease, Crohn's disease, collagen disease, tuberculosis, and malignancies appear to increase the demand for folacin (Exton-Smith, 1978).

Anticonvulsant drugs frequently used by the elderly are antagonistic to folacin. Research indicates that possibly 90 percent of all alcoholics are deficient in folic acid (Leevy and Kurnan, 1978; Halsted, 1980). This deficiency may be the result of liver damage or damage to the intestinal mucosa. Folacin is vital to the production of red blood cells. Without proper levels of folacin, macrocytic anemia occurs, a condition in which the red blood cells are larger and fewer in number than normal. Organic brain syndrome (OBS) has also been associated with low folacin intake (Batata et al., 1967). However, the nature of the relationship between the two is not clear. It is not known if the disorder leads to decreased dietary intake and a consequent folacin deficiency or if such a deficiency results in the impaired mental ability associated with OBS (Sneath et al., 1973).

Vitamin B_{12} is a compound which contains cobalt as a central part of its organic molecule. The exact functions of this vitamin are not completely understood. It appears necessary for cellular formation and functioning, especially in the bone marrow and digestive tract, and is needed to maintain the integrity of the nervous system. It is chemically interrelated with the vitamin folacin, is stored in the liver, and absorbed very slowly from the small intestine.

An intrinsic factor produced by the stomach is necessary for B_{12} absorption. If absorption does not take place, pernicious anemia results with its concommitant production of characteristically large, immature red blood cells. Vitamin B_{12}, as well as folacin, is needed for the maturation of red blood cells. When it is unavailable, these cells are pale, irregularly shaped, and reduced in number. Vitamin B_{12} absorption seems to decrease with age. This may result from a decrease in the intrinsic factor produced by the gastric mucosa. Antibodies against the gastric mucosa have been found in the blood of some patients, suggesting an autoimmune condition that may be responsible for disruption of the absorption of this particular vitamin (Davidson et al., 1975). Changes in gastric acidity, a malabsorption syndrome associated with partial or total removal of the stomach or ileum, and the taking of certain drugs can also interfere with the uptake of vitamin B_{12}. Deficiencies of this vitamin in the elderly are rarely due to low dietary intake. When B_{12} cannot be properly absorbed, it may be administered by injection.

A B_{12} deficiency may be associated with a folacin deficiency. In fact, suspected folacin problems should not be treated without first investigating vitamin B_{12} status. Folacin therapy can mask the earliest symptoms of B_{12} deficiency, delaying detection until irreparable nerve damage has been done. There is a possibility that a number of the elderly who are labeled "senile" or arteriosclerotic may have a B_{12} deficiency and suffer consequent alterations in brain functioning. It has been reported that some elderly persons who demonstrate confusion and disorientation show an alleviation of these symptoms when B_{12} is administered (Fleck, 1976).

As a component of coenzyme A, pantothenic acid is necessary to change fats and sugar into energy and is needed for the formation of adrenal and other hormones that also change proteins to fat and sugar. Some investigators (for example, Baker and Frank, 1968) have suggested that it plays an undetermined role in hypoglycemia. The vitamin is widely distributed in foods and no deficiency has been reported in human beings. Thus the elderly do not appear to suffer any special risks of a deficiency.

Vitamin C (ascorbic acid) is the only water-soluble vitamin not part of the B-complex group. Most species of animals are able to synthesize it from simple sugars, but man and his primate relatives must include an external source of vitamin C in their diet. Although vitamin C was the first vitamin synthesized in the laboratory, we still know very little about its specific chemical activity. Recently, vitamin C has been promoted as a cure or preventive for a wide range of conditions from the common cold to cancer. A number of exorbitant claims have been made about its therapeutic value. These claims have not been confirmed by carefully controlled scientific studies.

Vitamin C plays an important role in cellular metabolism but the mechanisms involved are poorly understood. Its most important function is in the formation and maintenance of collagen. Collagen forms the organic matrix of the connective tissue found in skin, bones, teeth, and muscle. The vitamin also plays an important role in wound healing and promotes elasticity and strength of capillary walls.

Vitamin C is important in folic acid metabolism as part of the reaction that converts folic acid to its active form, folinic acid. It also prevents the oxidation of folates, assuring their physiological activity. Vitamin C plays an important part in the absorption of iron from the intestine by reducing ferric iron to the more efficiently absorbed ferrous iron. Its role as an antioxidant, in the utilization of vitamin B_{12}, and in the body's detoxification process is not yet fully understood. The possible role of vitamin C in cholesterol metabolism and atherosclerosis must be investigated as well. Its role in the prevention of cancer has recently been challenged by a well-designed, carefully controlled double-blind study by Creagen and his associates (1979). The researchers found that among cancer patients the administration of 10 grams of vitamin C a day did not improve immune response or survival time.

The use of vitamin C to prevent the common cold has been the subject of controversy among researchers. Anderson (1972), in one of the best known and carefully conducted double-blind studies, concluded that vitamin C reduced the severity and frequency of colds. But he cautioned that the observed reduction might be due to a pharmacological rather than to a nutritional effect. To some researchers, it appears that vitamin C reduces the symptoms of a cold by an antihistamine effect, while at the same time leaving an individual's ability to transmit the disease unaffected (Anderson, 1972). Contradictory studies in this area necessitate more research and possibly better criteria for determining the presence or absence of "colds."

The role of vitamin C in the aging process may involve its relationship with vitamin E. It has been suggested that vitamin C synergistically aids vitamin E in antiperoxidative activities (Weg, 1978). At this time, there is little evidence to support this hypothesis. *Megadoses* of vitamin C may simply be a waste of money unless one is biochemically deficient in this vitamin. Toxicity from larger doses of vitamin C has not been a major problem, but side effects such as urinary tract stones (Stein et al., 1976), inactivation of vitamin B_{12}

(Herbert and Jacobs, 1974), and dependency deficiency have been reported (Rhead and Schrauger, 1971).

Vitamin C intake has been reported to be low in elderly populations, especially among those living alone or those who have disabilities that hinder shopping. Low serum ascorbic acid levels are not a normal accompaniment of biological aging, and the fact that older persons respond to supplementation seems to support this observation. The multiple stresses associated with aging, as well as some drugs, may depress vitamin C levels (Baker, 1967). Vitamin C is readily destroyed in food preparation and cooking and thus a marginal diet leaves little room for error. There is no reason to recommend an increase in vitamin C intake for the average older adult, unless future research supports higher RDAs of this vitamin for all ages groups. This increase has been suggested by Linus Pauling and his supporters, but rejected by most orthodox nutritionists.

MINERALS

Minerals are homogeneous inorganic substances that are necessary for the proper functioning of the body. Some of these minerals are referred to as macronutrients because they are needed in relatively large amounts (over 100 mg. per day). Others, needed in very small amounts, are termed micronutrients. Table 4.3 contains the 1980 RDAs and major dietary sources for minerals. The amount of a particular mineral needed in the body is not necessarily related to its relative biological importance. Each of these essential nutrients serves the body in one or more of five different ways:

1.   as a structural component of the skeleton;
2.   in the maintenance and regulation of the body's colloidal systems;
3.   in the maintenance of the acid-base equilibrium;
4.   as a component or activator of enzyme systems;
5.   as a component or activator in other biological units or systems.

Minerals are often interrelated in function and thus a deficiency of one may affect the functioning of others. For example, copper is necessary for the proper utilization of iron.

The degree of solubility of a mineral is generally related to its use in the body. Insoluble minerals are found in the teeth, bones, nails, and hair, while the more reactive minerals, such as the electrolytes, are found in the blood.

The absorption of most minerals by the body can be made very inefficient. A number of dietary, morphological, and physiological factors add to decreased absorption. The following factors have a tendency to reduce absorption:

1.   Chemical compounds, such as phytic acid and oxalic acid found in some foods (for example, spinach and oatmeal), combine with some nutrients such as calcium and iron to form insoluble compounds which are excreted.

2. High cellulose diets reduce the availability of absorption time by inducing hypermotility.
3. Laxatives and diarrhea can also produce hypermotility.
4. A deficiency or excess of one nutrient can reduce the absorption of another.

TABLE 4.3. RDAs and major dietary sources for minerals, 1980.

	MALES	FEMALES
Macronutrients		
Calcium (Ca)	800 mg.	800 mg.
Magnesium (Mg)	305 mg.	300 mg.
*Sodium (Na)	1,100–3,300 mg	1,100–3,300 mg.
*Potassium (K)	1,875–5,625 mg.	1,875–5,625 mg.
Phosphorus (P)	800 mg.	800 mg.
*Chlorine (Cl)	1,700–5,100 mg.	1,700–5,100 mg.
Sulfur (S)	No RDAs at this time	
Micronutrients (trace elements)		
*Manganese (Mn)	2.5–5 mg.	2.5–5 mg.
Iron (Fe)	10 mg.	10 mg.
Copper (Cu)	2–3 mg.	2–3 mg.
Iodine (I)	150 μ g.	150 μ g.
Zinc (Zn)	15 mg.	15 mg.
*Fluorine (F)	1.5–4 mg.	1.5–4 mg.
*Molybdenum (Mo)	.15–0.5 mg.	.15–0.5 mg.
*Selenium (Se)	.05–0.2 mg.	.05–0.2 mg.
*Chromium (Cr)	.05–0.2 mg.	.05–0.2 mg.
Vanadium (V)		
Cobalt (Co)		
Tin (Sn)	No RDAs at this time	
Nickel (Ni)		
Silicon (Si)		

Ca—milk, cheese, dark green leafy vegetables, legumes
P—milk, cheese, meat, poultry, grains
K—fruits, meat, milk, potato
Cl—salt
Na—salt, meat, cheese, processed food
Mg—whole grains, green leafy vegetables
Fe—eggs, meat, legumes, green leafy vegetables
F—drinking water, tea, seafood
Zn—meat, shellfish, nuts
Cu—meats, drinking water
I—iodized salt, marine products
Mn—legumes, cereals, nuts
Mo—legumes, meats
Cr—vegetables, whole grains

*Less information is available so the ranges are less precise and not as well graded by age.

Source: National Research Council, Food and Nutrition Board, 1980, *Recommended Dietary Allowances, Revised 1980.* Washington, D.C.: National Research Council-National Academy of Sciences.

5. Hypogastric activity due to antacid use or old age can reduce the solubility of all minerals.

In the elderly, mineral malnutrition may be related to decreased absorptive ability that comes with age, marginal diets, and to the effects of stress and immobilization in mineral balance. Next we will survey the major minerals that may be of significance to the elderly.

Calcium

Calcium is necessary for the proper mineralization of bone. It is important in the growth and maintenance of the skeleton and also plays an important role in blood clotting, cell wall permeability, muscle contractability, neuromuscular transmission, and cardiac function. The function of calcium is closely related to that of phosphorus and vitamin D. The ratio of calcium to phosphorus in the diet, which should be 1 to 1 and certainly not greater than 1 to 2, is crucial in determining the balance of calcium metabolism. If the phosphorus levels become too high, calcium is withdrawn from the bones to restore a proper equilibrium. Over the long term, this process can result in a gradual reduction of bone density.

Vitamin D aids calcium metabolism by enhancing transport of the mineral across the intestinal wall. Deficiency of this vitamin can result in disturbances of calcium metabolism known as rickets in the young and osteomalacia in the older adult. The body may be able to adapt to low intakes of calcium without immediate ill effects, but there is evidence that long-term low intake is undesirable since the amount of bone present in old age may be directly related to the integrity of the skeletal mass at maturity (Garn, 1975). Chronic nutritional imbalance during the twenties and thirties may affect the health of the skeleton in old age.

When a deficiency of calcium occurs, it is often accompanied by overly sensitive motor nerves, loss of muscle tone, and occasional decalcification of the bones. *Osteoporosis*, a decrease in total bone mass, is common in the elderly, especially females. Its cause has been attributed to the aging process, changes in hormone balance, long-term dietary practices, and physical inactivity. In the opinion of some researchers, the condition does not respond to calcium supplements (for example, Garn, 1975). However, calcium supplementation may still prove helpful in preventing further progression of the condition and bone resorption (Albanese, 1979). It has also been suggested that poor calcium intake may be a significant factor in the origin and progression of periodontal disease (Lutwak, 1976). There is some evidence that periodontal disease can be reversed by adequate calcium intakes (Lutwak, 1976).

There is no direct evidence of the necessity for increased calcium intake among the elderly. However, calcium intake can become deficient or imbalanced in older people due to chronic illness, malabsorption syndrome, increased lactase deficiency, and economic limitations. Chronic illness and malabsorption reduce the bioavailability of the mineral. The stress associated with both chronic illness and diminished psychosocial status can lead to increased calcium excretion as well as decreased appetite (Albanese, 1979; Watkin, 1979).

Phosphorus

Phosphorus is important in bone formation, metabolism and the transport of fatty acids. Phosphorus intake is frequently excessive among Americans who consume large quantities of meat and carbonated soft drinks while reducing their intake of dairy products. Excessive levels of phosphates in the blood are a threat to those of the elderly experiencing decreased renal function, and can be controlled by a diet high in carbohydrates and low in protein and phosphorus, or by use of an aluminum hydroxide gel to bind phosphorus in foods and the intestinal fluid (Watkin, 1979).

Magnesium

Magnesium plays an important part in cell respiration and the metabolism of fats, proteins, and carbohydrates. It is involved in the following functions:

1. bone and tooth formation;
2. muscle and nerve irritability;
3. delay in the formation of fibrin (necessary in blood clotting);
4. prevention of kidney stone formation.

Magnesium may lower cholesterol and retard lipid deposition in the aorta. A deficiency of magnesium is generally rare. Calcium/magnesium ratios may be more significant than the total level of magnesium. Reduced serum calcium levels are often present with magnesium depletion. Several complicating conditions common in the elderly can contribute to the production of a deficiency characterized by depression, muscular weakness, and convulsions (Shils, 1969). These conditions include chronic alcoholism, acute or chronic renal disease with defective renal tubular reabsorption, excessive use of diuretics, impaired gastrointestinal absorption, the use of certain antibiotics, and excessive use of enemas.

Potassium

Potassium is necessary for the maintenance of the body's acid-base and water balances as well as for proper neuromuscular function. Potassium deficiency can be a significant problem for the elderly. It is characterized by muscular weakness, disorientation, depression, and irritability. This deficiency becomes more common with age, especially among those on diuretics or those with prolonged diarrhea. Low potassium levels have been correlated with muscular weakness and some researchers suggest potassium supplementation as a course of treatment (MacLeod et al., 1975; MacLeod, 1975). Reestablishing a balance by dietary means can be difficult due to the frequently noted reluctance of the elderly to eat citrus fruits and milk. Bananas and apple juice seem to be more readily accepted and are good sources of potassium.

Sodium

Sodium, like potassium, is essential for water balance, acid-base equilibrium, and proper nerve function. A dietary deficiency of sodium is virtually unheard of in healthy adults. It can result from sodium restricted diets or diuretic therapy. A sodium deficiency can cause muscle cramps, mental apathy and reduced appetite. For most Americans, a deficiency of sodium is of less concern than is excess sodium intake.

Iron

Iron is needed for the formation of hemoglobin, and a deficiency of this mineral produces anemia. Iron deficiency anemia can cause fatigue, weakness, and listlessness, which if present add to the variety of factors reducing the quality of life for many of the elderly. To maintain an iron balance, an individual must absorb at least 1 mg. of iron per day to compensate for daily losses of iron in the shedding of cells even though the body recycles much of the heme from these shed cells.

Iron is converted to a form that is more absorbable by the activity of hydrochloric acid in the stomach. Many older individuals are subject to a reduced secretion of hydrochloric acid and a consequently reduced availability of dietary iron. Elderly people suffering from ulcers, malignancies, and hemorrhoids lose blood into the intestine and may develop an iron deficiency. Furthermore, many elderly people take aspirin or phenylbutazone which may cause internal blood loss.

Iron deficiency is difficult to treat by increased iron intake alone. Only an average of 10 percent of dietary iron is absorbed, and the absorptive potential varies from food to food. Consuming meat generally enhances iron absorption. Vitamin C and copper are necessary for the proper utilization of iron. Supplementation with ferrous iron may be necessary to meet the suggested daily intake of 10 mg. For the elderly on a low income, the daily intake of iron may be rather low given the expense of meats. In addition, fruits, which are a vital source of vitamin C, may similarly be avoided because of their high cost.

Zinc

Zinc is a component of several enzyme systems. It plays an important role in the synthesis of proteins and nucleic acids and is involved in insulin production. Deficiency in adults can result in poor appetite, an impaired ability for wound healing, and a diminished sense of taste and smell. Marginal zinc deficiency can be a problem in the elderly.

A number of conditions not uncommon in the elderly such as cirrhosis, kidney disease, malabsorption syndrme, malignancy, and alcoholism can promote a zinc deficiency. Some studies have suggested that healing and taste acuity improved after zinc supplementation. Since a relationship exists between zinc/copper ratios and hypercholesteremia, zinc supplementation must include a careful consideration of copper intake as well. It would, therefore, be wise for individuals of any age to avoid megadoses of zinc.

Iodine

Iodine is essential for proper thyroid function. Deficiencies do not appear to be a significant nutritional problem in the elderly. However, if an individual must go on a salt-free diet, alternative sources of iodine might be necessary. Many researchers believe that use of iodine in food processing has greatly increased the amounts supplied in U.S. diets (Mertz, 1981).

Fluorine

Fluorine has been linked to the prevention and treatment of osteoporosis. Its preventive role is probably established in early adulthood. Fluorine salts used in the treatment of osteoporosis can approach toxic levels and their administration should therefore be carefully monitored.

Chromium

Chromium is essential for the maintenance of normal glucose tolerance (Gurson, 1977). It may function as an insulin cofactor that serves to potentiate insulin by binding it to the cell membranes (Mertz, 1967, 1981). Chromium levels in the blood decline with age along with glucose tolerance. Some researchers have reported that chromium supplements for adult-onset diabetes improve glucose tolerance (Levine et al., 1968). Chromium may also be involved in controlling the level of blood lipids and the rate that lipid deposits accumulate in the aorta. Chromium supplements have been used successfully in older people to treat hypercholesteremia (Schroeder, 1976).

Selenium

Selenium is utilized by enzyme systems essential to the integrity of cell membranes. Selenium and selenium-containing amino acids may aid in preserving the stability of the membranes of such subcellular structures as the mitochrondia, microsomes, and lysosomes. Selenium appears to inhibit peroxidation, which can result in cell damage. It is possible that it works with vitamin E or at least serves to spare vitamin E in its antioxidant capacity (Li and Vallee, 1973). Thus a potential relationship between selenium and biological aging exists.

TABLE 4.4 Additional essential minerals.

MINERAL	FUNCTION
Copper	enzyme component essential for iron metabolism
Manganese	energy use (thiamine utilization) exotropic actions
Cobalt	constituent of vitamin B_{12} (dietary sources may be unnecessary since B_{12} is an essential nutrient)
Vanadium	mineralization of teeth and bones inhibition of a cholesterol synthesis may also have a toxic effect
Nickel	health of epithelial tissue
Molybdenum	prevent dental cavities iron metabolism
Sulfur	part of cell protein, cartilage and tendons detoxification process constituent of many proteins via S-containing amino acids
Chlorine	acid-base balance formation of gastric juice

Table 4.4 summarizes the possible functions of eight additional trace mineral nutrients that are significant in the overall consideration of an individual's nutritional pattern and requirements.

WATER

Water is one of the most significant components of a balanced diet at any age, though the elderly can be particularly vulnerable to water balance disturbances. All metabolic reactions require water, and sometimes even small changes in water balance can lead to metabolic irregularities.

Water is essential in a number of physiological functions. It aids the processes of swallowing, digestion and transport of ingested food, and is an important medium for waste elimination. It also functions in the regulation of body temperature through sweating and may aid in reducing the osmotic load on the kidney. In some geographic areas characterized by hard water, it can contribute to mineral nutrition by adding zinc, fluorine and copper to the diet.

Dehydration is not an infrequent occurrence in some elderly people. The condition may result from a disease and be exacerbated by minimal water intake. Dehydration can affect both fluid and electrolyte balance. The relationship of water intake to constipation and urinary problems will be discussed in Chapter 6.

Symptoms of water imbalance that are simply accepted as characteristic of old age can sometimes be controlled by carefully monitoring water intake. Water imbalances may result in such symptoms as apathy, body weakness, depression, mental confusion, and difficulty in swallowing. In order to maintain a proper balance of body fluid, water intake should be of sufficient quantity to produce a quart or more of urine per day. Nutritionists and physicians suggest the equivalent of approximately six to seven glasses of water a day to insure a proper water balance.

NUTRITION AND DRUGS

Nutrients and drugs interact in two major ways. First, drugs may have an effect on nutrient absorption and metabolism. For example, certain antibiotics lead to malabsorption of nutrients and a decrease in appetite. Second, the nutritional and health status of the host may affect drug metabolism. An example is the relationship between adequate protein intake and the potentiation of L-dopa in Parkinson's disease. These two kinds of interactions must be viewed against the declining ability of the aging organism to deal with the effects of some drug therapies.

Pharmacokinetics and pharmacodynamics provide specific information that is useful when considering interactions between nutrients and drugs. *Pharmacokinetics* concerns itself with how much, how long, when, how, if, and where a drug will be absorbed, transported, used, metabolized, and excreted (Poe and Holloway, 1980). *Pharmacodynamics* is the study of the biochemical and physiological effects of drugs and their mechanisms of action (Comfort, 1977). The study of pharmacokinetics and pharmacodynamics indicates that changes in drug utilization occur due to age-dependent factors.

Cardiovascular output decreases as one ages and thus can affect the distribution of pharmacological agents throughout the body. Gastrointestinal changes can reduce the absorption of drugs, and altered renal capacity affects the excretion of drugs. These observations necessitate the consideration of altered dosages and alternative drug choices and efforts to reduce multiple drug usage.

Roe (1976) has reviewed the evidence for the production of nutritional deficiencies during prolonged drug therapy. Elderly individuals and their health-care providers should be aware of the negative effects of uncompensated drug therapy and the impact of certain foods on the effectiveness of certain drugs. It should be remembered that the elderly, compared to the general population, take more drugs and are more likely to take multiple drugs and be chronic users of drugs (Lamy, 1980, 1981). They are therefore especially susceptible to drug-nutrient interactions. The problems, prospects, and theoretical models of drug nutrient interaction are complex and varied. An outline of the most important drug/nutrient interactions affecting the elderly is presented in Table 4.5.

SUMMARY

The six major nutritional constituents found in food sources are carbohydrates, fat, protein, vitamins, minerals, and water. These nutrients supply us with energy, aid in the growth and repair of body tissues, and help regulate body processes. Nutritionists continue to debate the specific amounts of each nutrient needed for optimal functioning. Included in this discussion is the concept of the recommended dietary allowances (RDAs). The RDAs are intended as reference points in planning diets to provide the greatest possible health benefits. They are revised approximately every five years.

The elderly have different nutritional requirements than do other age groups. Changes in digestive secretions, enzyme-producing organs, intestinal mucosa, and kidney functioning are examples of age-related physiological changes that affect how food is digested and nutrients are absorbed and excreted. Social factors also affect the nutritional requirements of older people.

The elderly represent special assessment problems for nutrition professionals. Changes associated with aging often imitate the signs of nutritional deficiency. Many symptoms of nutritional deficiency lack nutrient specificity. Diseases also alter the nutritional requirements of an affected individual.

Drugs and nutrients may interact in two important ways. The nutritional (and health) status of the individual may affect drug metabolism. Also, drugs themselves may have an effect on the way nutrients are absorbed and metabolized.

STUDY QUESTIONS

1. Differentiate between minimal and optimal nutritional requirements and indicate how they are related to the RDA concept.
2. In what ways can physical activity contribute to nutritional balance in elderly individuals?
3. What are the major problems associated with carbohydrate, protein, and fat consumption among the elderly?
4. Discuss the pros and cons of vitamin supplementation for the elderly.

TABLE 4.5 Nutrient/drug interactions to be aware of in elderly persons.

DRUG	NUTRITIONAL EFFECTS
Alcohol	Can lead to deficiencies in all nutrients, especially B vitamins. Can replace eating.
Aminopterin Methotrexate (used to treat leukemia)	Inhibits folate utilizations. However, if folate is supplemented, drug may not be as effective.
Antacids	Magnesium salts can cause diarrhea, limiting absorption of all nutrients. Protein absorption may be adversely affected when stomach acidity is reduced. Aluminum hydroxide binds phosphates.
Antibiotics	1. Tetracycline can bind iron, magnesium and calcium salts. 2. Many antibiotics are antagonistic to folic acid, and can result in deficiencies of other nutrients. 3. Can lead to malabsorption. 4. Neomycin binds bile acids and affects fat soluble vitamins absorption. 5. Neomycin causes intestinal structural changes that result in malabsorption of N, Na, K, Ca, lactose.
Anticoagulants	Can cause vitamin K deficiency.
Anticonvulsants	Primadone, phenobarbitol induce folate deficiency and vitamin D deficiency.
Antidepressants	Some cause accelerated breakdown of vitamin D. If the monamine oxidase (MAO) inhibitor-type is used, patients become intolerant to foods containing tyramine, such as aged cheese, red wine, beer, dry salami and chocolate. These foods can precipitate hypertensive crisis when MAO inhibitors are being used.

TABLE 4.5 (Continued)

DRUG	NUTRITIONAL EFFECTS
Aspirin and other anti-inflammatory drugs	1. Many cause gastrointestinal bleeding. Arthritic patients who ingest large quantities may develop iron-deficiency anemia secondary to blood loss. 2. Aspirin usage can affect folic acid status. 3. Aspirin and indomethacin can increase need for vitamin C by impairing its effectiveness.
Barbituates	1. Some cause breakdown of vitamin D. 2. Excessive sedation of nursing home patients for behavior control can result in missed meals. 3. Folic acid is malabsorbed.
Cathartics	Reduce intestinal transit time necessary for proper absorption of some nutrients
Cholesterol-lowering drugs such as chlofibrate	Any drug altering blood lipids can affect absorption of fat-soluble vitamins. Vitamin K deficiencies can be produced.
Colchicine, used in gout	Causes malabsorption of fat, carotene, sodium, potassium, vitamin B_{12}, folic acid, and lactose.
Diuretics	Most diuretics cause potassium to be lost in urine. Blood levels of potassium must be monitored, since mental confusion can result from low levels of potassium. Dietary sources of potassium should be consumed. (Magnesium may be deficient in long term diuretics.)
Glucocorticoids, used in allergy and collagen disease	Impair calcium transport across mucosa.

Hormones	1. ACTH and cortisone therapy increases excretion of sodium, potassium, and calcium, and may contribute to the development of diabetes, hypertension, obesity, and water retention. Calcium and potassium supplements may be needed, as well as special diet prescriptions if hypertension and diabetes develop. 2. Calcitonin treatment: decreases serum calcium levels as calcium is deposited into bone. Tetany may develop without oral calcium supplements. 3. Estrogen therapy: over an extended period, may result in deficiencies of folic acid and vitamin B_6. Patient should not receive folic acid supplements until vitamin B_{12} status is confirmed to be satisfactory. 4. Hormone therapy can cause peptic ulcers, which require dietary management. 5. Prednisone causes malabsorption of calcium.
Isoniazid (INH) (a drug used to treat tuberculosis)	Causes B_6 deficiency in some persons because it is an antagonist to the vitamin.
Laxatives	Harsh laxatives may cause diarrhea-like effects: food passes through the G-I tract too fast to be absorbed. Mineral oil absorbs vitamins A and D, preventing them from being absorbed.
Licorice candy	Limits potassium absorption.
Metformin and Phenformin Hypoglycemic agents Used in diabetics	Competitively inhibit vitamin B_{12} absorption.
Para-amino salicylic acid, used to treat tuberculosis	Can cause malabsorption of fat and folic acid. Blocks absorption of vitamin B_{12}.
Potassium chloride, used to replenish potassium lost due to diuretic use	Depresses absorption of vitamin B_{12}.

5. Identify the role and indicate some of the major problems among the elderly with regard to:
    A. Fat-soluble vitamins
    B. B-complex vitamins
    C. Vitamin C
6. What are the major functions of the essential mineral nutrients? Differentiate between macronutrients and micronutrients.
7. Why is the absorption of most minerals inefficient? Is this particularly significant for the elderly?
8. Identify the role and indicate the most significant problems among the elderly with regard to:

calcium	zinc	potassium	selenium
phosphorus	iodine	chromium	iron
magnesium	flourine	sodium	

9. Discuss the role of water and major problems associated with water imbalance among the aged.
10. Differentiate between pharmacokinetics and pharmacodynamics.
11. What age-dependent factors influence drug utilization?
12. Identify several drug-nutrient interactions that health care professionals need to be sensitive to among the elderly?

BIBLIOGRPAHY

ALBANESE, A. A., "Calcium Nutrition in the Elderly," *Nutrition and the M.D.*, 5, No. 12(1979), 1–2.

ANDERSON, T. W., et al., "Vitamin C and the Common Cold: A Double Blind Trial," *Canadian Medical Association Journal*, 107(1972), 503–508.

BAKER, E. M., "Vitamin C Requirements and Stress," *American Journal Clinical Nutrition*, 20(1967), 583–590.

BAKER, H. and O. FRANK, *Clinical Vitaminology: Methods and Interpretation*, New York: Wiley, 1968.

BAKER, H. et al., "Oral versus Intramuscular Vitamin Supplementation for Hypovitaminosis in the Elderly," *Journal of American Geriatrics Society*, 28, No. 1(1980), 42–45.

BATATA, M. et al., "Blood and Bone Marrow Changes in Elderly Patients with Special Reference to Folic Acid, Vitamin B_{12}, Iron and Ascorbic Acid," *British Medical Journal*, 2(1967), 667–669.

BRIN, M. and J. C. BAUERNFEIND, "Vitamin Needs of the Elderly," *Postgraduate Medicine*, 63, No. 3(1978), 155–163.

BROCKLEHURST, J. C. (ed.), *Textbook of Geriatric Medicine and Gerontology*. Edinburgh: Churchill and Livingstone, 1979.

CHERASKIN, E. et al., "Thiamin-Carbohydrate Consumption and Cardiovascular Complaints," *Internationale Zeitschrift Fuer Vitamin Forschune*, 37(1967), 449–455.

COMFORT, A., "Geriatrics: A British View," *New England Journal of Medicine*, 297(1977), 624.

CREAGAN, E. T. et al., "Failure of Dose Vitamin C Therapy to Benefit Patients with Advanced Cancer," *New England Journal of Medicine*, 301(1979), 687–690.

DAVIDSON, S., et al., *Human Nutrition and Dietetics*. London: Churchill and Livingstone, 1975.

EXTON-SMITH, A. N. and D. L. SCOTT, *Vitamins in the Elderly*. Bristol: John Wright and Sons, 1968.

EXTON-SMITH, A. N., "Nutrition in the Elderly," in *Nutrition in the Clinical Management of Disease*, J. W. T. Dickerson and H. A. Lee (eds.), Chicago, Year Book Medical Publishers, 1978.

FLECK, H., *Introduction to Nutrition*. New York: MacMillan, 1976.

FORBES, G. B. and J. C. REINA, "Adult Lean Body Mass Declines with Age: Some Longitudinal Observations," *Metabolism*, 19, No. 9(1970), 653-663.

GARN, S., "Bone Loss and Aging," in *The Psychology and Pathology of Human Aging*, R. Goldman and M. Rockstein, eds. New York: Academic Press, 1975.

GIRDWOOD, R. H. et al., "Folate Status in the Elderly," *British Medical Journal*, 2(1967), 670-672.

GURSON, C. T., "The Metabolic Significance of Dietary," in *Advances in Nutrition Research*, H. H. Draper ed. New York: Plenum, 1977.

HALSTED, C. H., "Folate Deficiency in Alcoholism," *American Journal of Clinical Nutrition*, 33(1980), 2736-2740.

HERBERT, V., "Biochemical and Hematologic Lesions in Folic Acid Deficiency," *American Journal of Clinical Nutrition*, 20(1967), 562-572.

_____, and E. JACOBS, "Destruction of Vitamin B_{12} by Ascorbic Acid," *Journal of American Medical Association*, 230(1974), 241-242.

HORWITT, M. K., "Vitamin E: A Re-examination," *American Journal of Clinical Nutrition*, 29(1976), 569-578.

LAMY, P. P., "Drug Interactions and the Elderly—A New Perspective," *Drug Intelligence and Clinical Pharmacy*, 14(1980), 513-515.

_____, "Nutrition and the Elderly," *Drug Intelligence and Clinical Pharmacy*, 15(1981), 887-891.

LEEVY, C. M. and T. KURNAN, "Nutritional Factors and Liver Disease," in *Modern Trends in Gastroenterology*, 5(1975), 250-261, London: Butterworths.

LEVINE, R. H. et al., "Effects of Oral Chromium Supplementation on the Glucose Tolerance of Elderly Human Subjects," *Metabolism*, 17, No. 2(1968), 114-125.

LI, T. K. and B. VALLEE, "Biochemical and Nutritional Role of Trace Elements," in *Modern Nutrition in Health and Disease*, R. S. Goodhart and M. E. Shils, eds. Philadelphia: Lea and Febiger, 1973.

LUTWAK, L., "Periodontal Disease," in *Nutrition and Aging*, M. Winick, ed. New York: John Wiley, 1976.

MACHLIN, L. J. and M. BRIN, "Vitamin E," in *Nutrition and the Adult Micronutrients*, R. B. Alfin-Slater and D. Kritchevsky, eds. New York: Plenum, 1980.

MACLEOD C. C. et al., "Nutrition of the Elderly at Home, III: Intakes of Minerals," *Age and Aging*, 4, No. 1(1975), 49-57.

MACLEOD, S. M., "The Rational Use of Potassium Supplements," *Postgraduate Medicine*, 57, No. 2(1975), 123-128.

MERTZ W., "The Biological Role of Chromium," *Federation Proceedings*, 26(1967), 186-193.

_____, "The Essential Trace Elements," *Science*, 213(1981), 1332-1338.

National Research Council, Food and Nutrition Board, 1980. *Recommended Dietary Allowances, Revised 1980*. Washington, D.C.: National Research Council - National Academy of Sciences.

POE, W. D. and D. A. HOLLOWAY, *Drugs and the Aged*. New York: McGraw-Hill, 1980.

RHEAD, W. J. and G. N. SCHRAUGER, "Risks of Long-Term Ascorbic Acid Overdosage," *Nutrition Reviews*, 29(1971), 262-263.

ROBERTS, H. J.,   "Perspectives on Vitamin E as Therapy," *Journal of American Medical Association*, 240, No. 2(1981), 129–131.

ROE, D.,   *Drug-Induced Nutritional Deficiencies*, Westport, Conn.: Avi Publishing Company, 1976.

SCHROEDER, H. A., "Nutrition," in *The Care of the Geriatric Patient*, E. V. Cowdry and F. U. Steinberg, eds. St. Louis: Mosby, 1976.

SHILS, M. E., "Experimental Production of Magnesium Deficiency in Man," *Annals New York Academy of Science*, 162, No. 2(1969), 847–855.

SNEATH, P. et al.,   "Folate Status on a Geriatric Population and Its Relationship to Dementia," *Age and Aging*, 2(1973), 177–182.

STEIN, H. B. et al.,   "Ascorbic Acid-Induced Uricosuria: A Consequence of Megaitamin Therapy," *Annals of Internal Medicine*, 84(1976), 385–388.

WALD N. et al., "Low Serum Vitamin A and Subsequent Risk of Cancer," *Lancet*, 2(1980), 813–815.

WATKIN, D. M., "Nutrition, Health and Aging," in *Nutrition and the World Food Problems*, M. Rechcigl, ed. Basel, Switzerland; S. Karger, 1979.

WEG, R., *Nutrition and Later Years*. Los Angeles: University of Southern California Press, 1978.

WHANGER, A. D.,   "Vitamins and Vigor at Sixty-five Plus," *Postgraduate Medicine*, 53, No. 2(1973), 167–172.

WILSON, E. D. et al., *Principles of Human Nutrition*. New York: John Wiley, 1975.

WINTERER, J. C. et al., "Whole Body Protein Turnover in Aging Man," *Experimental Gerontology*, 11(1976), 78–87.

YOUNG, V. R., et al., "Protein and Amino Acid Requirements of the Elderly," in *Nutrition and Aging*, M. Winick, ed. New York: John Wiley, 1976.

———, "Diet and Nutrient Needs in Old Age," in *Biology of Aging*, Behnke, J. A. et al, eds. New York: Plenum, 1978.

CHAPTER FIVE
THE BIOCULTURAL
BASIS OF GERIATRIC
NUTRITION

Aging is a biocultural process. Biology determines the potential duration of life, the relative length of the various phases of the life cycle, the physical signs associated with aging, and the nature and development of chronic and degenerative disease. Culture enables us to extend life expectancy through the development and application of science and technology. It also defines the stages of the life cycle and the ways in which people make the transition from one phase to another. Cultural stresses may even hasten the aging process.

There are two general but complementary approaches to a discussion of the biocultural basis of geriatric nutrition. The first involves the influence of nutrition on the biological aging process itself and its effect on the development of degenerative disease that often accompanies aging. A second approach is to examine the factors that influence the eating patterns of the elderly. The first approach was dealt with, in part, in Chapter 1 and will be further examined in Chapter 6. In this chapter, the second approach is emphasized.

SOCIOCULTURAL
FUNCTIONS OF FOOD

Food is necessary for an organism to survive and prosper physiologically. In humans, food and eating behavior are embedded in a *sociocultural matrix*. That is to say, in addition to biological nourishment, food serves many socially and culturally significant functions. These functions include the development of interpersonal relationships as well as feelings of security. Depending on the culture in question, food may also serve to express status, religious and/or ethnic identity, and feelings of pleasure and creativity.

Food influences behavior through *enculturation*, the process by which new generations come to adopt traditional ways of thinking and behaving (Harris, 1975). It is primarily based upon the control that older generations exert over the younger in terms of rewards and punishments. According to psychoanalyst Erik Erikson (1968), the first sustained human contact is the mother-infant relationship in which infant trust of the mother is learned as a function of the interaction associated with the feeding process. For older children, rewards and punishments may also involve food. Dessert may be offered or withheld in an attempt to influence behavior. For adults, certain types of food are used to gain social and economic advancement, to show conformity or rebelliousness, and to recognize important achievements. In our society, births, confirmations and bar mitzvahs, weddings, and even death may be "celebrated" with food.

Food is used to initiate and maintain a variety of interpersonal relationships. In fact, in most cultures, food is one of the most important means of fostering social relationships. Individuals can be held together or set apart by food and eating relations. Examples of the use of food in this way include coffee breaks and "brown bag" lunch groups at work or school, and community groups that share food and eat together at church or other gathering places. Generally, people share meals with friends, not strangers, though sitting down together for a meal is often symbolic of a truce between antagonists.

Food is important in the expression of group identify or solidarity. The former Catholic custom of abstaining from meat on Friday served as a group identification for those who adhered to it in the face of societal pressure to ignore church doctrine. Religious or supernatural ideologies often influence, even dictate, eating patterns. Eating or not eating certain foods or combinations of foods can demonstrate one's faith or serve as a protective device. Specific foods may serve as commemorative symbols recalling significant past events (for example, Easter or Passover). Among Eastern Orthodox Christians, lentil soup with vinegar is often served on Good Friday. The lentils are symbolic of the tears of the Virgin Mary, while vinegar reminds the faithful of Christ on the cross where he was given vinegar instead of water to drink.

Ethnic and/or racial identity can be reaffirmed by the use of traditional foods. The popularity of "soul foods" (for example, collard greens and chitlins) among northern Blacks is viewed by some as a return to cultural roots. The Black Muslim views this phenomenon quite differently and rejects "soul food" as symbolic of slavery, poverty, and degradation.

In part, people also eat for sensory pleasure. Taste, texture, appearance, novelty, and other organoleptic qualities may be the major reasons for eating or not eating certain foods. In the absence of other kinds of gratifications, special or forbidden foods may gratify those who are generally deprived in other ways.

Finally, food may serve to express an individual's creativity. The preparation of good or exotic food may be an individual's only recognized achievement. In such a case, food is a very important source of attention, status, and personal worth. Some individuals may exhibit creativity in food preparation in addition to other accomplishments. Such creativity may simply add to or enhance the individual's own perception of personal worth or increase his or her status in the eyes of others.

FACTORS AFFECTING NUTRITIONAL STATUS

The factors that affect the nutritional status of the elderly can be divided into two broad groups: (1) those which result from metabolic and physiologic changes associated with aging; and (2) those which affect the amount and type of food eaten. The latter group includes sociocultural factors, which are probably the most important influences on eating habits at any age. It also includes biological factors that can affect food selection and intake.

Affects on Metabolism and Physiology

It is generally recognized that caloric needs often decrease after age 55 (Winick, 1980). This results from decreased basal metabolism and a diminished activity pattern that is generally associated with aging. The slowing of basal metabolism is probably due to a loss of cell and tissue mass. Diminished activity may be a result of limitations brought on by chronic disease, lack of interest, or social isolation, among many other reasons. The topic of calorie imbalances resulting from age-related metabolic changes and activity diminution will be further discussed in Chapter 6 in a section on weight problems and aging.

The ability of the human body to respond to chemical imbalances is reduced with age. For example, after ingesting a dose of sodium bicarbonate, the body takes eight times longer at age 70 than it would at age 30 to reestablish normal sodium levels in the blood. There is some evidence of an age-associated decrease in the size and permeability of the capillary bed of the small intestine as well as a possible change in the permeability of the blood vessels as a result of collagenous changes. These alterations may diminish the capacity of blood vessels to take up and distribute nutrients (Exton-Smith, 1972).

Changes in digestive secretions may affect the digestion and absorption of food. The salivary glands begin to deteriorate at around age 60. This factor as well as certain others, such as "mouth-breathing," tends to dry the mouth, possibly forcing the selection of soft, self-lubricating foods. This in turn reduces the range of choice among foods and can result in a fiber-deficient diet that leads to or aggravates chronic lower bowel problems such as constipation. There is a decrease in the secretion of the intrinsic factor of the gastric mucosa which may be related to an age-associated decrease in the production of hydrochloric acid. This is significant because decreased intrinsic factor lowers the absorption of vitamin B_{12}, while reduced acidity affects iron and calcium absorption (Winick, 1980). There is a diminution of secreted pancreatic enzymes beginning at about age 40, but there are few hard data to indicate that age-related changes occur in the enzymes of the intestinal mucosa.

Age-related changes in the composition of the bacterial flora of the intestine have been documented. These changes can be detrimental, and are probably related to reduced gastric acidity or enzymatic action that allows the rapid growth of other organisms, such as streptococci, at the expense of the normal flora. This condition can result in the loss of nutrients synthesized by the displaced organisms as well as lowered resistance of the tract to disease. It also results in an irritated and inflamed mucosal lining.

Abnormal bacterial growth in the intestine can bind vitamin B_{12} and affect its availability for the body's use. Fat metabolism can be affected due to bile salt depletion resulting from bacterial deconjugation of bile salts. Further, some of the by-products of deconjugation may be toxic and/or carcinogenic to the gut. Occasionally, bacterial groups such as *Clostridia, Bacteroides* and *Veillonella* invade the small intestine from the large intestine, causing physical damage and upsetting environmental balances. This condition may necessitate short-term antibiotic therapy in conjunction with the administration of vitamins. In rare cases, when chronic conditions develop, intermittent long-term antibiotic therapy may be necessary.

Disorders of the hepato-biliary tract can also lead to fat maldigestion. This, in turn, can affect the body's utilization of the fat soluble vitamins A, D, E, and K. There is some evidence of a 20 percent reduction in lipolytic activity in the elderly, but this has no appreciable affect on fat digestion. Becker and his associates (1950) observed that it took aged individuals about twice the time required by younger people to absorb a high-fat meal.

Maldigestion and malabsorption are common conditions in the elderly, and the causative factors are numerous. These conditions, perhaps especially malabsorption, are responsible for many of the nutrient imbalances observed in the elderly. Balachi and Dobbins (1974) note some of the conditions that can lead to malabsorption. These include:

1. Surgical alterations (for example, esophagectomy, gastrectomy, and small bowel resections).
2. Pancreatic insufficiency caused by infammation or a tumor.
3. Hepatobiliary insufficiency caused by such conditions as gall stones and hepatitis.

4. Stasis and bacterial overgrowth.
5. Drug-induced changes caused by alcohol, anticonvulsants, cathartics, diuretics and antibiotics.
6. Cardiovascular abnormalities such as congestive heart failure, constrictive pericarditis, arteriosclerosis, and abdominal angina.
7. Radiation injury caused by accidental, occupational, or therapeutic exposures.
8. Endocrinopathy such as diabetes, Addison's disease, and thyroid disease.
9. Paget's disease.
10. Collagen vascular disease.
11. Amyloidosis.
12. Celiac disease, sprue.
13. Neoplastic disease.
14. Paraproteinemia such as multiple myeloma.

Malabsorption syndromes are difficult to manage when the small bowel mucosa are diseased. They can best be treated by parenteral administration of vitamins and minerals or the oral administration of pharmacologic rather than physiologic doses of these nutrients. Correction of the underlying condition should be the clinical goal, though this may be impossible since in many cases the cause of malabsorption is not known or the medical means to correct it are not available. In most cases of malabsorption, nutritional management is the only way of sustaining the patient. Any plan for its management must fit the individual case or circumstances.

Large-bowel problems are common concerns for many of the elderly. In particular, constipation or the fear of constipation has long been a concern for many older people. Even the casual observer might note the frequency with which advertising campaigns for laxatives are directed towards the elderly. Judging from the popularity of books on high-fiber diets (for example, Fredericks, 1976; Reuben, 1976; Galton, 1976), there is an increasing interest in the use of such diets. Recommendations for the use of high fiber diets seem to be related to an effort to prevent bowel cancer as well as a variety of other conditions, including hemorrhoids, diverticulosis, and diabetes. The clinical and epidemiological evidence supporting the widespread health benefits of a high-fiber diet is controversial and incomplete (Kelsay, 1978). Despite these inconclusive findings a great number of people have embarked upon preventive health programs based on increasing the amount of fiber in the diet.

Little evidence exists to suggest that significant amounts of essential nutrients are absorbed by the large intestine, but large intestine distress, real or perceived, can greatly affect the variety and nature of individual dietary choice, thus creating problems of imbalance. Many of these problems seem to be readily amenable to treatment if techniques of preventive medicine are used. Diet plays a significant role in preventive medicine, though dietary changes may be difficult to implement because of emotional attachments to long-standing dietary habits. However, the most efficient approach to most functional bowel problems is a therapeutic regimen consisting of dietary modification and increased physical activity.

Determinants of Food Intake

Those who work with the elderly often come to realize that metabolic and physiological barriers to proper nutrition may be minor compared to those factors that actually regulate food intake. Factors governing food intake determine the quantity, quality, and combinations of foods eaten, and are intricately interwoven into the fabric of the elderly person's social life. Again, food can be as important among the elderly for social and psychological reasons as it is for physiologic well being.

Biophysical and sociocultural variables affect food intake. The interaction of these variables results in a systematic process that affects both the biological and sociocultural environment of an individual to the aging process. Such adaption is truly biocultural in nature.

Biophysical changes that affect dietary intake include loss of teeth, reduced fine motor coordination, diminished vision, reduced sense of taste and smell, physical discomfort associated with eating, chronic disease, and decreased physical activity. These changes affect the efficiency of the alimentary tract and can alter dietary choice. They are also sometimes associated with changes in self-image as well as problems of isolation and depression. It is extremely important to remember that these conditions are not all "natural" and inevitable outcomes of the aging process. Many can be corrected or alleviated. For example, cataracts are the most common disability of the aged eye. It has been said that all of us would develop them, even if only to a mild degree, if we lived long enough. Those who have cataracts develop an opacity and frequently a yellowing of the normally transparent lens of the eye. The opaqueness of the lens interferes with the passage of rays of light to the retina. Depending upon the extent of cataract development, an individual will suffer a certain degree of blurred and dimmed vision. A person may need brighter and brighter light for reading and may also need to hold objects extremely close in order to be able to see them. Today, however, surgical removal provides safe and effective treatment for cataracts.

Loss of teeth or the existence of denture problems can lead to dietary modifications that stress foods which are softer and easier to chew. This can lead to reduced dietary bulk in the diet, further complicating lower bowel conditions, should they be present. Chewing problems of a mechanical nature are real for many of the elderly. Some studies have noted decreased efficiency in mastication with the successive loss of teeth. For example, the loss of a first molar can reduce efficiency on one side by as much as 33 percent (Neumann, 1970).

A denture wearer must chew food four times as long to reach the same level of mastication as a person with natural teeth. Half the population of the United States is in need of dentures by age 65 and about two-thirds are totally edentulous by age 75 (Busse, 1978). Well-fitting dentures do not exist since "fit" is a relatively subjective phenomenon that often depends on the adaptive qualities of the individual involved. It is easier to fit and satisfy younger old people in their 50s or 60s than the "old-old"—shrinkage of the gums and palate complicate the problems of fit for the very old.

Maxillary dentures usually fit better than mandibular dentures because of the broad-based structure of the maxilla. The greater mobility of the mandible and the tendency for the muscles and tongue to dislodge the denture during speech and swallowing make a comfortable fit in this area less likely. Public dislodgement of dentures can be embarrassing for sensitive individuals. Fear of such embarrassment can result in the rejection of nutritious foods to the detriment of the nutritional status of the individual.

The loss of neuromuscular coordination is a biophysical problem associated with aging. This condition can be further complicated by deteriorating vision, Parkinson's disease, stroke, or chronic arthritis. Fine motor coordination declines with age, but the existence of a chronic disease such as arthritis may greatly magnify the functional significance of any changes. Neuromuscular problems may lead to an inability to handle certain utensils, appliances, or foods. For those living alone, this inability can lead to the inefficient use of food resources. In the presence of others, both at home or in public, it is a source of embarrassment that can lead to a diminished use of important foods. The psychological effects of these reduced capacities and the situations they may precipitate can further diminish self-image and affect the social functions of eating. People who work with the elderly must be aware of these possibilities and try to suggest alternatives to insure adequate nutrition while preserving personal dignity.

A declining number of taste buds as well as neurologic problems can affect appetite. At age 70, there are only 30 percent of the number of taste buds present at age 30 (Arey, 1935). Loss of taste is a common complaint among the elderly. The ability to distinguish sweet, bitter, and sour tastes declines with age but the recognition of salty taste does not appear to be affected. (Hermel et al., 1970). Apparently, thresholds for each taste are not as affected as the ability to perceive subtle differences within each taste category. This may be problematic taken in combination with sociocultural factors that tend to suppress appetite. A diminished sense of taste can lead to overseasoning of foods with consequent irritation of sensitive parts of the digestive tract. In the case of salt, overuse can contribute to hypertension, heart disease, and kidney malfunction. No firm conclusion about the relationship between sensitivity to smell and aging can be drawn, although odor sensitivity seems to be very stable over age (Enger, 1977).

Most gastrointestinal discomfort associated with food ingestion is psychologically based, though biophysical causes such as hiatus hernia do exist. Useful research on the effect of particular foods on the digestive tract is scarce. If eating certain foods seems to induce symptoms such as heartburn and distension, elderly individuals should be encouraged to avoid them. Care must be taken to replace the nutritional contribution of the eliminated foods with alternative foods that are sources of the lost nutrients. Replacement is vital if an eliminated food was a key dietary source of essential nutrients. For example, if someone eliminates citrus fruit juice because it does not agree with him or her, care must be taken to assure proper vitamin C intake through consumption of alternative sources such as tomatoes and potatoes.

Chronic diseases also may necessitate modified diets. Chronic illness can deplete the energy needed to perform certain daily routines and affects motivation. Modified diets are often expensive and can be difficult to follow, especially if the person does not fully understand the necessity or the directions. Unfortunately, nutritional counseling is rarely available when this situation arises.

Elderly individuals can and must be made to realize the nature of their dietary problems. They should be educated to fully understand the regimen prescribed and the consequences of not following the regimen. An adequate counseling program consists of more than the providing of information on special diets. Diets should be devised to allow individual choice—monotony can destroy even the most well conceived diet.

Changes in the level of physical activity are also related to nutritional status. Exercise is needed to aid in the metabolism of foods. It is useful in relieving tension and maintaining mental well being and is necessary to maintain the strength and vigor to undertake everyday tasks. Lack of energy for shopping or meal preparation can lead to an undesirable emphasis on easily prepared, high-carbohydrate refined foods, such as bread, jelly, jam, or ready-to-eat cereals and cakes. Many of these foods have an extremely high sugar content. Mental stress from depression (and related inactivity) can lead to a further reduction in physical activity and consequently decrease energy and motivation necessary to shop for and prepare food.

The sociocultural factors that affect food intake are more varied and have a greater impact on nutrients than the biophysical factors discussed above. Each elderly person is the product of years of experience in a sociocultural setting modified only by individual perception and choice. Dietary habits and ideas are likewise longstanding and difficult to change. People often seem to arbitrarily prefer or reject certain foods in the face of direct evidence that such foods are good or bad for them.

The tendency to establish an attachment to certain foods may represent an individual's desire for security at a time in life when his or her level of insecurity, due to changing roles and status, is quite high. Dietary habits are often associated with memories of youth, pleasant and unpleasant, and in this context take on increased significance. Elimination of preferred foods or the addition of objectionable ones should not be attempted unless there is a definite threat to health. The psychological stress of such impositions can negatively affect the value originally associated with the dietary change.

Income is a primary factor in determining diet at all ages. Many gerontologists believe that the major problems of geriatric nutrition are a function not of age, but rather of the socioeconomic status of the aged. Our summary of the findings of recent national nutrition surveys (see Chapter 3) would suggest they are right. Retirement income, in comparison with preretirement earnings, is reduced for the great majority of older people. Poverty is a fact of life for many of the elderly, especially nonwhite aged (see Table 2.11). Housing, health care, transportation, and other expenses compete with money needed for food. Figure 5.1 shows the percentage distribution of average expenditures for families whose head-of-household is under 65 years of age as well as for families whose head-of-household is older. When compared with younger families, aged families spend a greater proportion of their income on food, housing, and health care.

Many elderly shoppers cannot buy food using the criteria of past eating habits or optimal nutrition because they possess insufficient purchasing power. They may develop a tendency to purchase cheaper foods that are high in refined carbohydrates, such as bread and cereals, rather than buying more expensive protective foods such as meat, fruit, and vegetables. It is not the carbohydrates per se that are bad, but rather the lack of dietary variety fostered by such purchasing patterns that often leads to reduced dietary quality and risk of malnutrition.

The elderly, like the poor in general, are often forced to shop at more expensive stores due to the absence of chain stores in local neighborhoods or lack of transportation to volume-sale stores with lower prices. Alternatively, the need to obtain credit to purchase food between retirement checks may arise. This necessitates the use of "Ma and Pa" grocery stores that give credit,

FIGURE 5.1. Percentage distribution of average expenditures, by age of family head: 1972–73. (Source: Herman B. Brotman, "The Aging of America: A Demographic Profile," in *The Economics of Aging, A National Journal Issues Book,* Washington, D.C.: Government Research Corporation, 1978, p. 38)

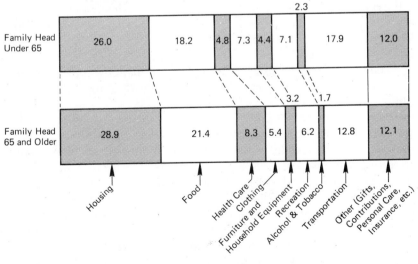

but must charge higher prices and carry a smaller variety of products than chain stores.

The elderly are often unable to take advantage of sales or quantity discounts because they lack proper storage facilities such as refrigeration and pest-free cupboards. Many people take for granted conveniences not always available to the poor or elderly. If money is not available for food at the time of the month when sales occur, the advertised bargains are unobtainable. Food activist groups have observed the deliberate price inflation of food products by food retailers at the time of the month when welfare and Social Security checks arrive. The poor certainly do pay more, and a significant proportion of the elderly are poor (Caplovitz, 1967).

Modern marketing procedures are geared toward the younger consumer with a family. The elderly need smaller quantities of food, especially those who live alone or have storage problems. Small quantities are often unavailable or, if available, are more expensive than the same foods bought in larger amounts. The current trend toward prepackaging perishables also creates problems for the elderly. The quantities prepackaged are aimed at families, not single consumers. This orientation makes it necessary, yet often embarrassing, for the elderly shopper to ask for less, which necessitates repackaging of the product. Furthermore, the packaging of food itself is a challenge to open, even for the young. Elderly individuals with failing vision, waning strength and declining fine coordination may be frustrated by such packaging materials. Marketing techniques aimed at higher profits such as end-of-aisle displays and multiple-item pricing affect both young and old. But many elderly have less margin for error in budgeting their limited funds.

As we have emphasized, eating is a social psychological activity (Pike, 1968). It is part of the complex arrangements of interpersonal interactions and, as such, has significant social and psychological impacts on the elderly. For the elderly, food can be a great comforter during times of loss, such as the death of a spouse or companion or the loss of social involvements. Losses force the rearrangement of the individual's world and upset balances. However, reestablishment of the old balance or creation of a new one may be difficult. Foods associated with significant events and periods in the lives of old people and their loved ones may be helpful in readjusting the individual's world.

Dietary stress can follow the loss of a spouse. Although widowers remarry at a substantially higher rate than widows, those of the elderly who do not may have special difficulty in adjusting. Widowers are often unable to take care of their own basic needs, especially if they have been married since youth and were socialized to depend heavily upon their wives. Because of this, some of the worst nutritional problems often occur among elderly widowers. Widows are able to continue to perform the domestic tasks that they have performed throughout their lives, but they may find themselves in financial distress. If her spouse had functioned as the money manager throughout the marriage, a new widow may be unable to cope with even simple household management problems. Even for those women prepared to handle these aspects of a spouse's death, the going may be difficult. Loss of companionship can seriously affect an individual's motivation to shop, cook, eat, remain active, or even go on living.

Loss of companionship may also reduce physical activity or social participation that previously diverted attention from many of the problems associated with old age. Emotional stress and depression are often associated with changing roles, isolation, chronic disease and disabilities, financial stress, and, simply, the fear of getting old. Depression is found in eight to 15 percent of those over 65 in the community and 50 percent of the 65 or older in nursing homes (Garetz, 1976). It may be associated with both over and undernutrition, either of which can lead to disability or death.

Emotional stress can cause a loss of appetite and the development of negative protein, calcium, and magnesium balances because of increased excretion often associated with stress (Altschule, 1978; Scrimshaw, 1964). Stress can also lead to compulsive eating and the onset of obesity which may further complicate health problems associated with old age. The elderly person who feels rejected or neglected by his or her family and friends may use eating as an attention-getting device. Others may not listen to frequent complaints about arthritis, but if a person is not eating or is eating too much, friends and relatives generally worry and pay more attention.

Isolation can affect motivation to eat, shop, prepare meals, and maintain social relationships. Many people can adjust to isolation if it is self-imposed and some may even prefer it. They may handle isolation well even when it is not self-imposed, if there is some hope of an eventual positive change in the situation. But few persons can manage isolation that is involuntarily imposed and which leaves them with no hope in sight.

Phillips (1957) has studied the relationship between losses, role changes, and adjustment to old age. His study of almost 1,000 aged individuals sixty and over—the retired compared to the employed, the widowed compared to the married—showed significantly more maladjustment in relation to old age. Maladjustment was measured by self-reports on the amount of time spent daydreaming about the past, thinking about death, and being absent-minded. Phillips argued that individuals who spend considerable time in such activities have difficulty in fulfilling their needs, including the need for appropriate caloric intake and dietary balance. Interestingly, Phillips employed a research variable he referred to as "identification as old." The item is a measure of self-image and simply asks, "How do you think of yourself as far as age goes—middle-aged, elderly or old?" He found that individuals who perceive themselves as elderly or old are significantly more maladjusted than those who perceive themselves as middle-aged. In addition, age identification appears to *reverse* the relationship between role loss and maladjustment. Thus, for example, those who are employed but identify themselves as old are more likely to be maladjusted than those who are retired but identify with middle age. How and why it is that some elderly individuals, even those who have suffered a role loss and are widowed, identify with middle age is still open to empirical investigation.

Finally, a number of basic logistical problems affect the ability of the elderly to get enough to eat. Lack of adequate cooking facilities may be a problem for those living in low-cost housing such as rented rooms or single-room-occupancy hotels. The use of cooking facilities may be discouraged by the presence of appliances or utensils that are old or dangerous. Pots with loose or absent handles and dull can openers can cause painful burns or cuts for an elderly person with poor vision or coordination problems. One solution to such minor environmental threats is avoidance, though losing the option to use such devices may seriously limit the range of possibilities for meal preparation and nutritional intake.

FOOD FADDISM

The dangers of food *faddism* are a subject that nutrition educators tend to overwork or exaggerate. The large majority of people who engage in food faddism—patronizing health food stores or stocking up on megavitamins—do not have their health threatened, but simply pay more for what they eat (Metress, 1980). It is often alleged that the elderly are particularly susceptible to the promises of food faddism. Although no empirical attempt has been made to ascertain whether the effects of food fads are positive or negative, most standard sources simply assume a negative impact.

If, indeed, the elderly are more susceptible to food faddism, what are the possible reasons and what are the possible effects on health? The attitude of organized medicine toward aging and geriatric problems may play an important role in the popularity of geriatric food faddism. With minor exceptions, modern medicine, which still emphasizes acute, curative care, has shown little interest in geriatric medicine. For many physicians, the problems of elderly patients are seen in terms of a negative prognosis. In this regard, physicians mirror the values of our society as a whole with regard to aging.

Given this situation, it is not surprising that many elderly people turn to food fads. The fad gives the individual at least what appears to be some authoritative sanction for what are, many times, false hopes. However, at least the individual can feel that he or she is actively doing something about his or her condition, and not just passivly allowing it to deteriorate.

Poor nutrition education during younger years also affects an individual's ability to evaluate nutritional claims. Without accurate knowledge, the consumer (at any age) is easy prey for flashy, manipulative advertising pitches by both food faddists and corporate producers. According to Gussow (1978), the deficiencies in current nutrition education in America are due to poorly trained health educators, government neglect, and corporate control. We have been socialized to "a quick-fix mentality" (Metress, 1980). Americans seem to be constantly searching for simplistic technological solutions to societal problems of all types. Socially and psychologically, food fads represent an example of a falsely simplistic solution to fears and doubts about health and aging.

Many basic nutrition textbooks have made reference to the harmful effects of food faddism on the health of the elderly (for example, hypervitaminoses). Is there really a threat, and if so, is it of minor or major proportions? Certainly, a variety of harmful effects can occur. These include vitamin toxicity, complication of existing health conditions, delay in seeking needed treatment, undue expense, unbalanced diets, and simple disappointment. But what are the realities of these threats to the well-being of the elderly?

Toxicity due to superintake of some nutrient is a common charge of critics of food faddism. A review of the literature, however, discloses no quantitative and little anecdotal evidence of toxicity due to food fads among the elderly. Actually, the two best known threats of hypervitaminosis involve the fat-soluble vitamins A and D. Given the fat malabsorption problems often associated with the aging gut, it seems unlikely that enough of either of these vitamins would be absorbed to lead to hypervitaminosis in most cases (Metress, 1980). However, the threat of complications in existing conditions is real. Occasionally, radical diets aggravate a pathological state such as constipation or diabetes, or can cause gall bladder trouble. Most people have some awareness of the limitations imposed by their known medical problems. However, undiagnosed threats could pose a problem for the fad eater, but the necessary coincidence of pathology and fad is probably rare.

Self-treatment with fad diets could delay securing necessary medical treatment and this delay is, perhaps, the most serious consequence of all self-care strategies. Most serious disorders, however, are of such a nature as to cause alarm in a person despite attempts to deal with it through self-care. The undue expense of adherence to self-treatment regimens has been advanced as another negative effect, especially for those on marginal incomes. The costs of the fad may divert needed money elsewhere—this would seem to be a real concern.

The threat of unbalanced fad diets leading to the possibility of covert or even overt malnutrition would not seem to be a significant concern except for those on an extreme dietary regimen. To date, there is no evidence that elderly people suffer from such dietary deficiencies due to this factor. Finally, the disappointment that false hope brings is more often short-lived than not and is certainly of no great long-term psychological significance for most people. The concept and consequence of false hopes is relative to a particular situation. A so-called false hope may lead to better adjustment to a condition for which little can be done anyway.

Are there benefits in the practice of food fads? If so, do they outweigh the possible threats? This is a difficult question to answer empirically. Some food fads may actually have beneficial effects or at least lead to better eating habits. With regard to the recent revival of interest in fiber as an important constituent of the diet, it must be recalled that for years this nutrient was also promoted by food faddists.

Participation in faddism may result in a psychological lift related to the feeling that at least one is doing something about the "miseries" of old age. This kind of psychological uplift may motivate some to resume activities that were given up or curtailed. Increased participation can lead to a renewed interest in life and the development of a more positive attitude toward the self.

NUTRITION EDUCATION
AND THE ELDERLY

The standard approaches of nutrition education can rarely compete with clever advertising aimed at profit-making and unrelated to good nutrition. Most advertising is geared to selling a product, not nutrition, and it often contains negative nutrition messages coupled with a lack of accurate information. Some advertising techniques are solely created with the psychological manipulation of the consumer in mind.

Nutrition educators have become overdependent on the *Basic Four* food group model in teaching choice. Recent studies at the University of California at Berkeley have revealed that the basic four planned diet met the RDA for only eight out of seventeen nutrients required daily (King et al., 1978). Using the basic four model, a poor diet may be selected unless the individual has access to the knowledge of the nutrient value of foods in *each* group. Many foods available today do not fit into the basic four groups because they are mixtures or fabricated products. In addition, the basic four model was developed before RDA's existed for vitamin E, B_6, folacin, B_{12}, phosphorus, magnesium, iodine, and zinc. The model is just vague enough to permit the possibility of nutritional detriment. For example, using the basic four model, one could select a diet that is characterized by improper nutrient ratios, outright deficiency of some essential nutrients, and filled with potentially dangerous additives. A newer, more functional approach is needed, based on factual knowledge about individual foods, how they are processed and marketed, and their possible contribution to individual health and well-being (Graubard, 1944). Nutrition education should be geared to geographic location, cultural variation, socioeconomic disparity, and educational level. It must be approached with dignity and with consideration for the experience and social image of the elderly. Older people want sound information and will respond positively to interesting approaches that utilize this information.

The popularity of well written pseudoscientific nutrition literature can be taken as a gauge of the public interest in this topic. If journalistic popularizers of nutrition can interest the public in their nutritional message, why are nutrition professionals unable to do the same?

mixtures of fabricated products. In addition, the basic four model was

Education programs that detail health and consumer protection problems can be useful in combating nutritional misinformation and deceptive advertising. This effort is worthy, but difficult. The monopolistic food industry, with its large advertising budgets and product development research, has considerable access to the American people, and comparable influence.

Print and electronic (radio, TV) media materials geared to the elderly of different levels of income and education are needed. The former should be effectively arranged in a concise manner with relatively large type so that it can easily be read by those with failing vision. In both forms excess verbiage should be avoided and care must be taken to arrange the message in a logical, easily understood progression with examples when necessary. Information should be of a practical nature with an allowance for a variety of food patterns related to such factors as economics, ethnic background, and religion. In certain regions of the country, the availability of such information in a multilingual format is essential.

SUMMARY

Aging is affected by the interaction of biology and culture. Biology determines the potential duration of life. Culture enables us to extend life expectancy through the development and application of science and technology. Nutrition is also a biocultural phenomenon. Food is necessary for an organism to survive and prosper physiologically, yet it also serves many socially and culturally significant functions. Food may be useful in the development of interpersonal relationships and may help express feelings of security, economic status, religious and/or ethnic identity, and feelings of pleasure and creativity.

Factors that affect the nutritional status of the elderly can be divided into two broad groups: (1) those that are the result of metabolic and physiologic changes that accompany aging, and (2) those that affect the amount and type of foods eaten. The first group of factors are principally biological and biophysical while the latter group includes sociocultural factors.

Sociocultural factors that affect food intake are more varied and have a greater impact on choice of nutrients than biological and biophysical factors. Among these sociocultural factors are dietary habits associated with youth and security, income, place of residence, living arrangements, and marital status.

Though based on speculation, it is generally believed that the elderly are particularly susceptible to food faddism. Food fads often give the individual pseudo-authoritative sanction for his or her beliefs in false claims about extending life expectancy or reducing the risk of disease. Current nutrition education in America leaves most consumers both old and young unable to evaluate exaggerated nutritional claims. However, participation in a food fad may still give an individual a psychological lift in a perceived battle against old age.

STUDY QUESTIONS

1. Why is aging a biocultural process?
2. What are the two general but complementary approaches to the discussion of the sociocultural basis of geriatric nutrition?
3. What are the major sociocultural functions of food?
4. Discuss the effects of age-related changes in metabolism and physiology on the nutrition of the elderly.
5. Identify the major age-related biophysical changes that affect the intake of food among the elderly.
6. Identify the major sociopsychological changes that affect nutritional intake in the elderly.
7. Identify the major socioeconomic changes that affect nutritional intake in the elderly.
8. Discuss the possible impact of food faddism on the elderly.
9. What are some of the major problems associated with nutrition education that can affect efforts to communicate with the aged consumer?
10. Why can we refer to nutrition as a biocultural system?

BIBLIOGRAPHY

ALTSCHULE, M., *Nutritional Factors in General Medicine.* Springfield, Illinois: C. C. Thomas, 1978.

AREY, L. B., "The Numerical and Topographical Relation of Taste Buds to Human Circumvallate Papillas Throughout the Life Span," *Anatomical Record,* 64(1935), 9–25.

BALACHI, J. A. and W. V. DOBBINS, "Maldigestion and Malabsorption: Making Up for Lost Nutrients," *Geriatrics,* 29(1974), 157–160.

BECKER, G. H. et al., "Fat Absorption in Young and Old Age," *Gastroenterology,* 14(1950), 80–92.

BROTMAN, H. B., "The Aging of America: A Demographic Profile," in *The Economics of Aging, A National Journal Issues Book,* Washington, D.C.: Government Research Corporation, 1978, p. 38.

BUSSE, E. W., "How Mind and Body and Environment Influence Nutrition in the Elderly," *Postgraduate Medicine,* 63(1978), 118–125.

CAPLOVITZ, D., *The Poor Pay More: Consumer Practices of Low-Income Families.* New York: Free Press, 1967.

ENGER, T., "Taste and Smell," in Birren, J. and Schaie, K. (eds.), *Handbook of the Psychology of Aging.* New York: Van Nostrand Reinhold, 1977.

ERIKSON, E., *Identity, Youth and Crises.* New York: W. W. Norton & Co., Inc., 1968.

EXTON-SMITH, A., "Psychological Aspects of Aging: Relationship to Nutrition," *American Journal of Clinical Nutrition,* 25, No. 8(1972), 853–859.

FREDERICKS, C., *Carlton Fredericks' High-Fiber Way to Total Health.* New York, Pocket Books, 1976.

GALTON, L., *The Truth About Fiber in Your Food.* New York: Crown Books, 1976.

GARETZ, F. K., "Breaking the Dangerous Cycle of Depression and Faulty Nutrition," *Geriatrics,* (1976), 31:6:73–75.

GRAUBARD, M., "Nutrition Education in Labor Organizations," *Applied Anthropology,* 3(1944), 26–37.

GUSSOW, J. D., "Thinking About Nutrition Education: Or Why it's Harder to Teach Eating than Reading," Paper presented at AAAS Meeting, Houston, January 6, 1978.

HARRIS, M., *Culture, People, Nature: An Introduction to General Anthropology.* New York: Thomas Y. Crowell, 1975.

HERMEL, J. et al., "Taste Sensation Identification and Age in Man," *Journal of Oral Medicine,* 25(1970), 39–42.

KELSAY, J. L., "A Review of Research on Effects of Fiber Intake in Man," *American Journal of Clinical Nutrition,* 31(1978), 142–159.

KING, J. et al., "Evaluation and Modification of the Basic Four Food Guide," *Journal of Nutrition Education,* 10, No. 1(1978), 27–29.

METRESS, S. P., "Food Fads and the Elderly," *Journal of Nursing Care,* 13(1980), 10–13, 24.

NEUMANN, G., *Lectures in Bioanthropology.* Indiana University, Bloomington, Indiana, 1970.

PHILLIPS, B., "A Role Theory Approach to Adjustment in Old Age," *American Sociological Review,* 22(1957), 212–217.

PIKE, M., *Food and Society.* London: John Murray, 1968.

REUBEN, D., *The Save-Your-Life Diet.* New York: Ballentine, 1976.

SCRIMSHAW, N., "Ecological Factors in Nutritional Disease," *American Journal of Clinical Nutrition,* 14(1964), 114–122.

WINICK, M., *Nutrition in Health and Disease.* New York: John Wiley, 1980.

CHAPTER SIX
NUTRITION, DISEASE, AND DISABILITY

Nutrition has been implicated as a factor in a variety of disease and disability conditions. However, scientists do not always agree on the nature and significance of various nutritional factors, and thus alternative theories of disease etiology arise. The source of much of this disagreement is often methodological. Many nutrition-related diseases are difficult, if not impossible, to develop for study in ordinary laboratory animals. In addition, it takes years for such diseases to manifest themselves in humans. Conditions such as coronary heart disease, maturity-onset diabetes, and bowel cancer are usually characterized by a long latent period making longitudinal research problematic.

Much of the evidence now available on the relationship between nutrition and aging and disease is of an epidemiological nature. In some cases the epidemiological studies are not supported by experimental data. Statistical correlation between diet and disease may represent a positive association but does not "prove" causality. Future research must collect, analyze, and integrate experimental and epidemiological data in order to test the various diet-disease hypotheses extant today.

This chapter will attempt to present a brief overview of disease and disability conditions associated with the aged that have a significant dietary component. While these conditions are not exclusive to later adulthood, a significant proportion of the elderly people are affected by them. Some result from the interaction of nutritional status with the normal biological aging process, while others result from the interaction of nutrition and disease.

SKIN CONDITIONS AND
THE SKELETOMUSCULAR
SYSTEM

Decubitus Ulcers

Decubitus ulcers are sometimes referred to as bed or pressure sores. Those at highest risk for the development of these sores are the nonambulatory elderly. Some believe that the absence or presence of pressure sores is actually an indicator of the quality of nursing care being delivered. Prevention, then, is the most significant part of decubitus ulcer care. The nutritional component of a preventative approach is not insignificant as both obesity and underweight increase the risk of occurrence. Adipose tissue is poorly supplied with blood vessels and thus more susceptible to bed sores, while wasted individuals have an inadequate cushion against boney prominence pressure. Pinel (1976) has observed that anemia lowers oxygen content of tissue and encourages tissue necrosis; Michocki and Lamy (1976) found that 45 percent of those with decubitus ulcers were anemic. Thus it would appear that some form of iron supplementation would be helpful in preventing the condition.

Osteoporosis

Osteoporosis has been accepted as a natural phenomenon of aging and, like arteriosclerosis, is found almost universally in the elderly, although it can occur at any age. The condition takes years to develop, but often manifests itself quite suddenly and painfully. It is the result of a gradual loss of bone that reduces skeletal mass without disrupting the proportion of minerals and organic materials distributed throughout. This quantitative loss of bone mass can result in diminished height, slumped posture, backache, and a reduction in the structural strength of the bones, making them more susceptible to fractures.

Osteoporosis can involve most of the bones of the skeleton, but most disability and pain is due to vertebral osteoporosis. Although the majority of affected individuals do not have a demonstrable pathology, bone loss is severe enough to cause fracture in at least 30 percent of the cases (Lutwak, 1969). As a result of its largely asymptomatic development, the prevalence rate is difficult to determine, but estimates vary from 10 to 50 percent of those over 50 years old in the United States (Avioli, 1977). There are differences between men and women in the rate and degree of bone loss, with the incidence and severity being more pronounced in women. Weg (1978) suggests that one-third of the women over 60 are affected, while Smith and Rizek (1966) estimated that 50 percent of the postmenopausal women in the U.S. are affected. Albanese and colleagues (1975) found its incidence four times higher in women and determined that this difference increases with advancing age. Men do develop osteoporosis, but not as early or as severely as women.

Osteoporosis can be classified into two categories, primary and secondary. Causes of the condition such as cortiocosteroid excess, hyperparathyroidism, and renal failure explain secondary osteoporosis, but less is known about primary osteoporosis. Several theories have been formulated to explain its etiology. Among the factors proposed as having a significant role in the development of primary osteoporosis are: (1) decreasing activity levels; (2) reduced absorptive efficiency of the aging gut; (3) reduced renal resorption; (4) decreasing neural impulse leading to the loss of muscle and bone together; (5) hormonal changes with age; (6) hereditary predisposition; and (7) dietary deficiency. The following discussion deals with the contribution of diet to the development of primary osteoporosis.

Gender differences in incidence and severity have led to the association of adult bone loss with menopause and ensuing estrogen deficiency. However, Garn (1975) counters that more bone loss occurs than can be accounted for by an estrogen-withdrawal theory. Loss often continues long after the cessation of menopause, and the condition does occur in men. Researchers disagree on the value of hormone therapy employing supplemental estrogen. The possible relationship of estrogen replacement therapy to breast and uterine cancer also raises a serious question of risk-benefit for those opting for the treatment (Recker et al., 1977.)

The observed incidence of seemingly excessive osteoporosis in women may be the result of a number of factors. The bone mineral reserves in young women are threatened by the impact of sex-exclusive phenomena such as dieting and child birth. Dieting is dually stressful. Weight loss "promotes" bone loss, and reducing diets are notorious for being nutritionally imbalanced. Related to child-bearing is the possibility that lactation may deplete bone mineral reserves—up to 300 mg./day of calcium must be provided by the mother to nourish a newborn infant. Hormonal changes at menopause also tend to accelerate bone loss. When these factors are added to the longer life expectancy of women, a clearer picture emerges as to why women are at greater risk for developing primary osteoporosis.

Inactivity has also been cited as a major cause of bone loss, but quantifying the actual effect of exercise on bone development and maintenance is difficult. It is known that bone and muscular activity are important in stimulating osteoblastic activity and that immobilization can induce significant osteoporosis (Whedon, 1980). Genetic factors are not completely understood either, but may play a significant role. For example, blacks in general have denser bones than whites; hip fractures are 10 times more common in white women than black women (Bollet et al., 1965).

Specific dietary elements such as calcium-phosphorus ratios, protein, vitamin D, vitamin C, and fluoride have been implicated by a number of researchers (Lutwak, 1976; Bullamore, 1970; Jowsey, 1976; Ellis et al., 1972). Calcium deficiency has long been included in explanations for osteoporosis, but more recent studies indicate that disease-onset may not be related to immediate or recent calcium intake (Lutwak, 1976). Increased fecal loss of calcium with advancing age has been noted and may be due to age-related changes in the efficiency of intestinal absorption and possible increase of lactase deficiency. At the same time, calcium intake tends to decrease with age (Odland et al., 1972). These observations have led some to conclude that negative calcium balances are more likely in older persons. However, calcium supplementation in old age has not yielded impressive results. The calcium intake hypothesis is not supported by studies of individuals who have a high intake of the mineral, although a history of low calcium intake is often noted in those with severe osteoporosis (Lutwak, 1976). A recent study by Smith's (1976) research team indicates an association between low calcium intake and higher fracture rates at all ages.

In Guatamala, native people with diets low in quality protein and high in calcium had a bone loss rate similar to Americans who had a high protein, low calcium intake (Garn, 1975). It appears that the amount of bone present at maturity may be most important in the development of adult bone loss. Actual amount of loss may be influenced by heredity, disease stress, endocrine activity, and physical activity as well as intake levels of calcium and other essential nutrients.

Many researchers feel that a chronic deficiency of calcium accompanied by a chronic excess of phosphorus during the growing years may be significant in the development of osteoporosis (La Flamme and Jowsey, 1972). An imbalanced ratio of calcium and phosophorus in contemporary diets has been noted in the U.S. where high meat and soft drink consumption result in high phosphorus consumption. Lutwak (1976) suggests that this chronic imbalance leads to steady demineralization of the skeleton beginning at age 20. Further, he argues that modern diets exhibit 1:4 calcium/phosphorus ratios while the optimum ratio appears to range from 2:1 to 1:1.

A high rate of protein consumption has also been implicated in osteoporosis since there are indications that as protein levels increase, calcium levels must also increase in order to maintain equilibrium. Kim and Linksweiler (1979) report that increased protein intake causes increased calcium resorption from bone. Thus long term consumption of a high protein diet with low calcium intake can increase the risk of osteoporosis. Schuette and his colleagues (1980) found that a high protein diet increases calcium excretion. This conclusion was confirmed by Licata and colleagues (1981). Linksweiler (1974) observed that calcium/protein equilibrium was possible with an intake of 400 mg. of calcium a day and 42 gm. of protein a day. When protein levels were raised to 95 to 142 gm. a day there was a reduction of calcium retention and the development of a negative calcium balance. A daily loss of 100 mg. of calcium could result in significant loss of bone over a 10 to 20 year period. Even a loss of 30 mg. a day over 20 years could result in a loss equivalent to 1/3 of the total skeleton.

Another theory proposes that meat-rich diets have caused acid overloads which in turn produce calcium loss. There is little "hard" data to support this theory, although Barzel (1970) found improved negative calcium balances in subjects receiving sodium and potassium bicarbonate in capsular form. Some studies among Eskimos (who are heavy meat eaters) indicate that bone loss for both sexes is 5 percent greater per decade than observed in the United States (Mazess and Mather, 1974, 1975).

Some researchers claim that a vegetarian diet can decrease bone loss. Studies of long time vegetarians indicate that their bone density is greater than that of omnivores and they are less likely to develop osteoporosis (for example, see Ellis et al., 1972). Also, bone density showed significantly less decrease with age in vegetarians and the decreases did not continue after age 69 as in omnivores. These studies have been challenged on methodological grounds. Challengers cite the small and unequal number of subjects in study groups, the lack of information on the duration of time subjects followed their dietary regimens, and the problems of radiological interpretation that often confuse bone density and photographic density.

Lutwak (1969) has suggested that the dietary fat content of a diet may affect calcium absorption. In the presence of excess fat (150–200 gms./day) and at levels less than 50 grams/day, calcium absorption is impaired. It appears that the optimum level of fat intake in relation to calcium absorption is 100 to 125 grams a day.

Vitamin C and D have also been implicated in osteoporosis development by some researchers. Vitamin C plays a role in collagen synthesis but at this time the extent of its involvement in osteoporosis is relatively unknown. Vitamin D deficiency leading to a fall in calcium absorption and retention after the age of 70 has been noted by Bullamore and his associates (1970). Liver disease, kidney disease, and gastric surgery may interfere with the metabolism and absorption of vitamin D and produce the symptoms of deficiency. Albanese (1976) has noted that therapy consisting of 750 mg. of calcium along with 375 international units of vitamin D daily stopped bone loss and increased density up to 12 percent. Slovik and his team (1981) have recently demonstrated the impaired responsiveness of 1, 25-dihydroxy vitamin D production as a result of the infusion of human parathyroid hormone fragment 1-34 in older patients. They suggest that deficient secretory reserves of 1, 25-dihydroxy vitamin may explain the inability of older patients to adapt to low calcium diets characteristic of old age. In another recent study Gallagher (1979) suggests that impaired vitamin D metabolism may be related to an observed decrease in calcium absorption with age.

Fluorine seems to increase the formation of new bone as well as the crystallinity of bone material. Populations from regions with fluorine-rich water do not appear to have as great a risk of osteoporosis as those from other regions (Bernstein et al., 1966). Jowsey (1975, 1976) has noted some improvements in bone mass and some reversal of osteoporosis when a combined regimen of fluoride, calcium, and vitamin D supplementation was utilized. The exact nature of this complex interaction is not understood. The fact that too much flouride in the presence of diminished calcium can lead to both osteoporosis and osteomalacia urges some caution on this issue.

As has already been indicated, dietary treatment of osteoporosis has not been an unqualified success. However, a recent study by Lee and his team (1981) reports on a diet intervention study with elderly women that resulted in increased bone density. The diet combined calcium-rich foods with calcium supplementation. At the Mayo Clinic a supplementation program that includes calcium, vitamin D, and fluorine has been reported to increase new bone formation, though there is some question as to the bone's structural adequacy. Targovnik (1977) and Albanese (1976) had some success with combined calcium/vitamin D supplements but noted little or no improvement in the first 6 to 9 months. In some circumstances a long period of dietary supplements may be necessary to achieve significant results. In a more recent report, Albanese (1979) suggests that a daily intake of 1200 mg. of calcium may be of benefit to the elderly. Jowsey (1975, 1976) has argued for the combined use of calcium, fluorine and vitamin D once osteoporosis is discovered to be present.

Osteomalacia

Osteomalacia is often confused with osteoporosis, but is characterized by defective mineralization rather than a decrease in total bone volume. Defective mineralization may result from a failure of the process of mineralization or because mineralization takes place at a slower rate than the formation of new matrix. There are more than thirty causes of this condition, most of them rare, but basically it is due to an imbalance of calcium, phosphorus, and vitamin D.

Dietary osteomalacia rarely occurs in the United States today, but it is found among those who have undergone gastric surgery. It has been noted frequently in individuals with femoral neck fractures and can be confused with Pagets disease or with a fracture callus. The symptoms usually include weakness, pain, disability, and skeletal fractures or pseudo fractures known as Looser's zone. Table 6.1 presents a clinical comparison of osteomalacia and osteoporosis. Differentiation between these two conditions is extremely important since the treatment for osteomalacia is highly effective, unlike that for osteoporosis.

Although osteomalacia is not an overwhelming problem for the aged in the United States, a few age-related changes relative to this condition deserve attention. It is possible that the intestine may absorb calcium less efficiently with advancing age so that more vitamin D and calcium may be needed. In addition, changes in the skin that accompany aging may effect the efficiency

TABLE 6.1.   Comparison of osteomalacia and osteoporosis.

OSTEOMALACIA	OSTEOPOROSIS
1. Muscle weakness	1. No muscle weakness
2. Poorly localized skeletal pain and tenderness	2. No skeletal pain and tenderness
3. Frequent painful rib fractures	3. None
4. Large amounts of uncalcified bone matrix	4. Normal degree of calcification
5. Pelvic deformity common	5. No pelvic deformity
6. Peripheral bones more marked	6. Axial bones more marked
7. Looser's zone present in radiographs	7. Looser's zone not present
8. Abnormal values for serum calcium, inorganic phosphorus, serum alkaline phosphatase	8. No biochemical abnormalities

with which vitamin D is synthesized. Chalmers' research group (1967) found a number of their patients who indicated a diminishment of symptoms in the summer months.

A possible major risk in the treatment of osteomalacia in the United States involves interaction with other medications. For example, aluminum antacids, used by many of the elderly on a long-term basis, have a tendency to bind phosphorus. Likewise, anticonvulsant drugs such as phenobarbital can inactivate vitamin D metabolites, thus causing a vitamin D deficiency. Dietary deficiency of vitamin D, however, is not considered a common cause of osteomalacia. It would appear that limited exposure to sunlight and malabsorption problems (for example lack of bile or pancreatic disease) are more important in the development of osteomalacia. For example, in hepatic disease more vitamin D may be required since a liver enzyme converts the vitamin to its active form. Treatment for osteomalacia is usually simple and very effective and consists of supplements of vitamin D and calcium. The amount and nature of supplementation depends on the etiology and severity of the condition.

Osteoarthritis

Osteoarthritis is a degenerative joint disease in which there is a gradual wearing away of joint cartilage during the process of aging. Pain and stiffness can result from exposure of underlying bone surfaces, but inflammation is generally absent. Weight-bearing joints in long-standing osteoarthritis often become unstable or disorganized (Kart et al., 1978).

The cause of this disease is obscure, but its incidence is significantly correlated with age (Lawrence et al., 1966). Although there is no cure, symptomatic relief can be achieved. Drug therapy and regimens to reduce joint strain have proven to be effective in many cases. From a dietary perspective, a program to reduce weight or at least maintain weight at a desired level can help relieve joint pain and stress and prevent more extensive damage to affected areas. Also, it is important to be aware of the nutritional risk associated with obligatory drug therapy. Aspirin therapy, used to relieve pain, has been associated with blood loss and iron deficiency anemia, and vitamin C deficiency can manifest itself through cutaneous bleeding. Steroid therapy can result in bone demineralization, sodium retention, negative nitrogen balance, and edema. Machtey and Quakmire (1978) reported that over 50 percent of a small sample of elderly people showed some improvement of symptoms after a daily dose of 600 mg. of vitamin E.

Rheumatoid Arthritis

Though rheumatoid arthritis affects fewer people than osteoarthritis, it is more serious and can lead to greater disability. The condition may start at any age, and most often adults carry it with them into old age. The cause of rheumatoid arthritis is unknown, though it is commonly referred to as an autoimmune disease (see Chapter One).

As a chronic, inflammatory disease that is two or three times more common in women, rheumatoid arthritis can lead to a great deal of pain, discomfort, and disability. Aspirin is a mainstay of therapy for this condition and carries with it risks of iron deficiency anemia, vitamin C deficiency, and peptic ulcer. Steroid use presents the same problems referred to in the discussion of osteoarthritis. An appropriate diet would prevent a negative nitrogen and calcium balance that could lead to muscle atrophy and decalcification of bone. Since many rheumatoid arthritis sufferers are underweight, a weight reduction program is not as important as it is in osteoarthritis.

Gout

Gout is a genetic disorder of purine metabolism. It is characterized by excessive levels of uric acid in the blood due to either increased production and/or faulty elimination. Sharp salt crystals (urates), precipitated out to the joints, initiate attacks resulting in sudden, excruciating pain, swelling, and inflammation. The role of these salt deposits is not yet understood. Anti-inflammatory drugs and drugs that lower uric acid levels are part of the therapy.

At one time it was believed that excessive eating and drinking of rich foods and alcoholic beverages brought on the manifestations of gout. Such suppositions are now being questioned. Since gout represents disordered purine metabolism, foods high in purines should be restricted. However, a restricted purine diet does not always guarantee decreased blood levels of uric acid. Purines can be manufactured by the body from simple metabolites.

Hence, uric acid levels can increase even though outside purine sources are being controlled through dietary restrictions.

However, some general dietary recommendations are still in order for persons with the ailment. Fats, proteins, and carbohydrates are all necessary in a balanced diet, but excessive amounts of fat should be avoided by the gout sufferer since they prevent the excretion of uric acid. Protein intake should not be excessive, but a substantial number of calories derived from carbohydrates helps to increase uric acid elimination. Fluids should be increased to aid acid excretion and minimize the risk of renal calculi formation.

During the acute stages of gout, it is best to severely restrict purine intake to avoid increasing the already high levels of uric acid in the blood. Foods high in purine include meat gravies, broths, bouillons, consommés, organ meats, anchovies, mackerel, herring, sardines, scallops, mussels, and sweetbreads. Food allergies have been known to instigate gouty arthritis and, for this reason, gout sufferers would do well to stay away from any foods to which they are allergic.

Persons with gout, often obese, should never go on rapid weight-loss diets. Weight-loss increases uric acid levels and creates a metabolic state similar to that seen in a high-fat diet. Use of diuretics can actually induce attacks of gout. Therefore, it is extremely important that weight-loss occur at a gradual rate, and that such a diet never be initiated during an acute attack.

NEUROSENSORY DISEASE: PARKINSON'S

The most common movement disorder involving the central nervous system among the elderly is Parkinson's disease. It develops later in life, usually the sixth decade, and is more common in men than women. Rigidity, tremors, slowness of movement, and drooling affect the afflicted. Also occurring may be poor grip, sucking deficiency, reduced hand-to-mouth coordination, and a much-limited ability to bite, chew, and swallow, all of which make self-feeding difficult. Weight loss can be beneficial since many of the symptoms are aggravated by obesity. Modified eating utensils with built up handles, spouted cups, and plate guards on rims are also helpful (Mitchell et al., 1976). Levodopa, or L-dopa, represents a recent advance in drug therapy for Parkinson's disease. This synthetic drug effectively raises levels of dopamine, which is present in insufficient amounts in untreated patients. Its action serves to prevent dopamine destruction and to reverse or reduce many of the symptoms of Parkinson's disease such as muscle rigidity, postural problems, speech disorders, and tremors. Patients who are on L-dopa therapy should not take multiple vitamins containing vitamin B_6 (pyridoxine), which interferes with the therapeutic effect of the medication. Likewise, they should reduce their protein intake since L-dopa is an amino acid and competes with other amino acids for intestinal absorption (Sweet, 1975).

NUTRITION AND ORAL HEALTH

Dental Caries

Dental caries, or tooth decay, is the greatest cause of tooth loss up to age 35, but subsequently periodontal disease becomes the greatest source of tooth loss. However, dental caries still continues to be present, and the effects of earlier dental caries persist in the form of missing teeth and the use of dental plates in later years.

Three factors are present in caries production: (1) a more or less susceptible tooth, (2) bacterial plaque on the surface of the tooth, and (3) a dietary substrate such as carbohydrates. A variety of oral bacteria is capable of causing tooth decay, but the major culprit appears to be streptococcus mutans, which readily ferments monosaccharides and disaccharides to lactic acid.

The process of tooth decay starts with the formation of a sticky viscous film called plaque in which bacteria grow, multiply, metabolize food debris, and convert carbohydrates to organic acids. The plaque protects the bacteria of decay from normal oral cleansing. Organic acids, such as lactic acid, make contact with the tooth enamel and demineralize tooth hydroxyapatite. This, in turn, allows the bacterial proteolysis of tooth collagen, creating cavities. The amount of decalcification and decay seems to be related to the length of time cariogenic bacteria are in contact with the tooth.

Prominent in the decay process is sucrose, which is involved in three ways. It is easily converted by bacterial enzymes to dextrans and levans which form the structural basis of plaque. Second, in the plaque itself, it serves as a reserve food supply for bacteria that remains available even after all traces of a meal have disappeared from the oral cavity. Finally, sucrose itself is readily converted by bacterial action to lactic acid.

The role of saliva in the process of tooth decay is still unclear. It has been suggested that it helps clear food residues and neutralizes the acid medium essential for decay. Urea in the saliva may be converted to ammonia by ureolytic microbes in the plaque resulting in a higher pH. Others have suggested that saliva may serve as an ionic source of flourine, calcium and phosphorus, all of which are incorporated into the tooth surface structures.

It is difficult to determine the effects of specific nutrients on caries development. Tooth resistance is a developmental phenomenon, so an earlier nutrient imbalance may affect resistance to decay later in life. A number of nutrients have been implicated in the process of tooth decay. Among them are protein, fats, phosphates, a variety of trace elements, and simple carbohydrates. Protein may protect against tooth decay by increasing the salivary urea and ammonia levels to neutralize the pH, promoting an immune response that may inhibit bacterial colonization and generally assuring the integrity of body tissues. Fat seems to have cariostatic effects such as increasing anti-microbial activity, reducing time and quantity of food retention on teeth, increasing flow of saliva, and aiding in the production of a protective film on the teeth (DePaola and Alfano, 1977).

It is possible that phosphates cleanse the teeth and aid in remineraliza-tion of tooth surfaces. The calcium to phosphorus ratio may also be related to caries development. Mann (1962) found a calcium/phosphorus ratio of .55 to be associated with few or no caries. A number of other trace elements—molybdenum, strontium, vanadium, lithium, barium, and boron, are described as cariostatic, while lead and selenium have been associated with cariogenesis (Glass, et al., 1973). The systematic effects of most of these trace elements on tooth resistance are still unclear.

Flourine has been shown to influence caries development through a variety of mechanisms that are still not fully understood. Its ingestion during tooth development can reduce caries by 60 percent, while topical applications after eruption can lead to reductions of 20 percent (DePaola and Alfano, 1977). In one way, flourine appears to be related to the formation of a stabilized enamel apatite that resists dissolution by organic acids. In another, it may be related to the promotion of recrystallization of carious teeth. Some flourine ions seem to replace hydroxide ions in the apatite (fluoroxyapatite), forming an acid insoluble matrix that is fixed for the life of the tooth. It may also affect the efficiency of plaque formation or the capacity of some microbes to break down sugars to acids.

Dietary supplements in the form of flouride tablets are apparently not practical as they are rapidly cleared from the body, and it is hard to deliver the exact amounts needed physiologically. Flourine added to salt at the level of 90 mg. of flourine per kilogram of salt can result in a 30 to 40 percent reduction in decay. At present, flouride is added to water supplies throughout the United States and is most effective at levels of 0.7–1.2 parts per million (ppm) of drinking water. Levels about 1.5 ppm can result in discolored or mottled teeth. While flourine and phosphorus appear to be cariostatic, selenium, magnesium, cadmium, lead, silicon, and platinum have been reported as caries-promoting. Also, deficiencies of vitamin C, zinc, and protein may increase the pathologic potential of oral bacteria by allowing easier penetration of the teeth by bacterial toxins.

Simple carbohydrates have been strongly implicated in the promotion of tooth decay. The form of the sugar and the length of retention in the mouth appear to be more important than the amount. The physical consistency of a food is related to retention and hence cariogenic potential; solid foods are worse than liquids, and sticky foods such as carmel, sweet pastry, ice cream, and syrups are the most troublesome. The circumstances surrounding con-sumption also play an important role. For example, sugar at mealtime or with liquids is less cariogenic than between meals. It has also been suggested that sugary foods containing phosphates are less of a threat because of the cariostatic influence of phosphates.

General advice concerning diet and dental decay should include the elimination or reduced use of cariogenic foods and the addition of possible caries-protective foods such as fats and proteins, and the inclusions of foods that require strong mastication. Evidence that other sweeteners help reduce caries incidence is unclear and conflicting.

Although caries constitute a less serious problem in later years, prevention of the condition should be a significant part of health maintenance among the aging. Previous caries experience determines the number and quality of teeth caried into old age, and the maintenance of healthy teeth should continue. The number and condition of the teeth affect the efficiency of the digestive process and can influence dietary intake. Also, the presence of healthy teeth is important for the anchorage of a partial dental plate, which is functionally preferable to a full plate.

Periodontal Disease

As indicated earlier, periodontal disease is the leading cause of tooth loss after age 35. When only the gums and soft tissues are involved, the condition is referred to as gingivitis, but when bone is also affected, it is called periodontitis. Systematic factors involving hormones and nutrition as well as plaque formation are important in its etiology (Bahn, 1970). The process of periodontal deterioration is initiated by bacterial action in the gingival crevices. Plaque develops, causing one of the most concentrated bacterial populations known to affect human beings. The gum margins fall away from contact with the teeth, and the process invades the bone, eventually affecting the periodontal ligament which can lead to tooth loss. Chronic infection associated with this process can also lead to tooth loss.

Nutritional status affects an individual's susceptibility to periodontal disease. It may exert its influence by promoting an immune response, enhancing tissue integrity, and affecting the production of saliva and gingival fluid. Tough, fibrous foods may be effective in removing plaque. Tough foods also help minimize gland atrophy and encourage increased saliva flow with a higher protein content (Alfano, 1976) though there is a little conclusive evidence at this time that saliva actively deters periodontal disease.

As a caries development, soft sticky carbohydrate foods are an effective medium for bacterial growth, especially beneath the gum margin. This can obviously contribute to more optimal subgingival conditions that are possibly related to plaque formation and periodontal involvement. Fibrous foods, however, increase keratinization of the epithelial tissue, making it less susceptible to attack.

Calculus or tartar, a hard deposit of calcium salts, mucin and bacteria, is also associated with periodontal disease. The cause of tartar formation is obscure, although it may simply be an advanced form of plaque. It appears that the massaging effect of rough food prevents its formation.

Lutwak (1976) has suggested that periodontal disease may be, in part, a form of nutritional osteoporosis, the dietary factor being a chronic dietary deficiency of calcium in association with excess dietary phosphorus. American diets are notably high in phosphorus due to the large amounts of meat, poultry, fish, milk, and flour consumed. Milk consumption has generally been declining in the American diet, and it has often been replaced by soft drinks that are notably unbalanced in their calcium/phosphorus ratios. As evidence, Lutwak (1976) cites retrospective studies that link the appearance of vertebral osteoporosis and periodontal disease, and severity of axial osteoporosis and edentulousness. Clinically, evidence that calcium supplementation can do more than halt the progress of osteoporosis has not been produced. But, from a preventive point of view, proper calcium/phosphorus ratio should be stressed for dietary intake during the earlier adult decades. This will allow individuals to proceed into middle and old age with a healthy periodontal bone structure. An optimally developed skeletal structure can possibly slow the onset and reduce the severity of age-related periodontal bone disease, more so than a skeletal system that is already in precarious balance.

THE AGING
GASTROINTESTINAL TRACT

Hiatus Hernia

Hiatus hernia can lead to a number of esophageal symptoms or complicate other existing conditions. There are basically two types of hiatus hernia: the common sliding type and the paraesophageal type. In the common sliding type, the junction of the esophagus and the cardiac portion of the stomach move above the normal position at the diaphragm and lead to gastric reflux. In the paraesophageal type, a portion of the cardiac end of the stomach herniates through the diaphragm hiatus alongside the esophagus. Sometimes a third type is identified, which is the result of a congenitally short esophagus and causes the same symptoms as a hiatus hernia. This third type is really not a hernia, although it is sometimes accompanied by a sliding hernia.

Hiatus hernia appears to be increasing in incidence, and the majority of affected individuals are over 50 years old. Women appear to be affected more than men. In an early study, Brick and Amory (1950) observed it in only 18 percent of their subjects below the age of 50 but in 28 percent of those over age 70. McGinty (1971) noted that hiatus hernia occurs in possibly 65 percent of those over 60 and most often in obese women.

Hiatus hernia can occasionally lead to complications such as esophagitis and ulceration and stricture of the esophagus. Surgical correction is rarely recommended and usually has a slim chance of success. Medical management such as weight reduction, changes in the size and frequency of meals, medication, and sometimes sleeping with the head of the bed elevated is usually sufficient to obtain relief.

Cholelithiasis (Gall Stones)

Gallbladder problems are a major source of concern and stress for many elderly people. The incidence of these problems increases markedly after age 65 and generally coincides with changes in the ability of the gallbladder to empty and alterations in the physical composition of bile. Bertolini (1969) found that bile tends to be thicker, richer in cholesterol, and reduced in volume in the elderly. Statistics reflect the increase in the incidence of gallstones with age. Somewhere between 15 percent and 33 percent of those over 70 are afflicted by gallstones. Ponka's research group (1963) found that 55 out of 200 aged patients with abdominal pain had gallstones (cholelithiasis). Stones are more common in elderly women than men, but after age 70 sex differences are insignificant. Those with diabetes, on estrogen therapy, and with bile absorption problems have an especially high risk of developing gall stones. Most cases in the elderly appear to be asymptomatic, though common manifestations include indigestion, nausea, vomiting, fat intolerance, obstructive jaundice, and episodes of cholecystitis.

Lack of bile in the small intestine can lead to deficiencies of the fat-soluable vitamins. As a precaution, persons with a gall bladder condition should receive vitamin K supplements prior to surgery. However, the course of treatment for gallstones is debated by surgeons. Some prefer surgery even if the person is asymptomatic, in an effort to forestall such complications as a ruptured gallbladder or carcinoma. Others believe that a more conservative approach with emphasis on medical management is the best source of action. This latter attitude is based on the increased risks that surgery present, the fact that the incidence of carcinoma of the gallbladder is low, the possibility that other diseases or conditions may be causing the symptoms, and the general mental stress imposed upon an elderly patient by surgery. Medical treatment usually consists of a program of weight reduction, avoidance of fatty foods, and the use of antacids.

Liver Disease

Cirrhosis of the liver is final and most serious stage of liver injury and degeneration. The liver is in a contracted state and loses most of its ability to function, and once a fibrous connective tissue replaces the liver cells, cirrhosis is irreversible. It is the ninth most common cause of death in the United States today and is positively associated with chronic alcoholism, which itself is an all too common occurrence in the elderly.

The nature of the relationship between cirrhosis and alcoholism is still being debated. One current view holds that cirrhosis is a result of the interaction of chronic alcoholism and long-term nutritional deficiencies from which most alcoholics suffer. Such deficiencies can lead to a fatty liver and cause its eventual fibrosis. The liver becomes more susceptible to damage from toxic agents and infectious organisms when nutritional deficiency is present as well.

Diet is an important aspect in the treatment of cirrhosis. A diet high in calories using mainly carbohydrate and protein sources with moderate amounts of fats and provisions for appropriate vitamins, is the best regimen for maximum recovery. It allows for the repair of hepatic cells and supports hepatic function. Vitamin supplements and liver extract are often recommended. Protein should be rich in lipotrophic factors, which mobilize liver fat and thus act to prevent fatty infiltration and degeneration of the liver cells. Since the appetite of a patient with cirrhosis is often poor, six to eight small meals a day would be most effective.

Diverticulosis

Diverticular disease of the colon tends to be a disease of the later decades of life, increasing in occurrence from age 40 onward. It appears to be increasing in incidence, especially in the industrial nations. In 1900, diverticular disease was practically unknown in the western world. In the past 75 years it has become the most common affliction of the colon. It may affect over a third of the population over the age of 50 in the industrial countries, but it is unknown or rare in most developing countries. Women appear to be affected more often than men, and the overall number of diverticula increase with age. The most common site of this condition is the sigmoid colon. McKeown (1965) found the incidence of diverticulosis with symptoms to be about seven percent in those over 70 while Berman and Kirsner (1972) observed the condition in 40 percent of those over 70, but symptoms can range from none at all to peritonitis.

Diverticula are actually tiny herniations of the mucous and submucous layers through the muscle layer. They form a pocket or balloon-like structure that projects from the bowel about one to two centimeters. Fecal matter can collect at the opening of a diverticulum and form fecoliths, which ulcerate the mucosa and promote infection. The symptoms of diverticulitis are abdominal pain, diarrhea, constipation (or alternating bouts of each), and bleeding. Complications are rare, but on occasion diverticula can perforate and give rise to pericolic abcess, peritonitis, or fistula of the bladder, vagina, or other parts of the gut. These conditions call for immediate surgery.

In general, medical management may consist of a high-residue diet and antibiotic therapy using septrin, neomycin, or phthalylsulfathiazole. The use of a high-residue diet is a complete therapeutic turnabout from the previous treatment, which called for a bland, low-residue diet. Painter and Burkitt (1971) showed that adding bran to a diet as a fiber supplement gave good results in treating diverticular disease.

Burkitt (1978) has proposed that diverticular disease, along with gallstones, hiatus hernia, adenomatous polyps of the large bowel, varicose veins, appendicitis, carcinoma of the large bowel, ischemic heart disease, and even obesity can be associated with a highly refined diet that is short of dietary fiber. Indigenous African populations eating higher fiber diets have a rapid transit time for food passage through the gastrointestinal tract and large, soft stools. In the case of industrial societies, this is not so—transit times are three to seven days compared to a little over thirty hours in Africa, and stool weight averages 100 grams a day as compared to 300 grams in Africans. Burkitt believes that viscid feces are more difficult to propel, thus raising the pressure within the lumen of the intestine and forcing the pouches of the intestine out through weak spots in the muscle layers to form diverticula. At this point, the weight of the evidence seems to support the Burkitt hypothesis, but one should be cautioned against attempting to view fiber diets as a "miracle cure-all."

Hemorrhoids

Hemorrhoids are present in most people over 50 years of age. They consist of ruptured blood vessels that are located around the anal sphincter. They can be either external or internal, and they can be asymptomatic or very painful with bleeding that necessitates surgery. Some of the major causes in the elderly are constipation, prolonged use of cathartics or enemas and straining on the stool. Dietary treatment can make a bowel movement movement comfortable and promote healing. In general, eight to 10 glasses of water a day and a diet that is balanced but bulk-producing can reduce or prevent hemorrhoids. The use of harsh laxatives should be avoided, and the time of bowel movement regularized each day. The increased incidence of hemorrhoids in the Western world has also been related to a low-fiber diet.

Constipation

Many elderly people worry constantly about constipation, but there is no evidence that it is an inevitable outcome of aging. The causes of constipation are varied, ranging from lack of exercise, overuse of cathartics, and psychological stress to gastrointestinal disease or an unbalanced diet.

Many elderly people today were raised during a time when a daily bowel movement was considered to be essential for good health. Perhaps this fixation on regularity will abate as the currently younger generations become older, although the interests of the pharmaceutical and advertising industries are in keeping this myth alive. Few serious attempts have been made to determine the range of variation in frequency of human bowel movement. A number of researchers believe that age-related frequency in laxative use may be obscuring related changes that do occur (Connell et al., 1965).

In treating constipation, an individual approach is most efficient. After the possibility of disease or obstruction has been ruled out, a therapeutic regimen consisting of dietary modification and increased physical activity should be worked out. For instance, fiber included in the diet may help increase water-holding qualities leading to bulky stools that are more easily excreted. Dietary changes, however, are difficult to implement, since long-standing food habits often hold great emotional significance. Physical exercise, too, may be a difficult therapy to implement.

More than 700-over-the-counter constipation remedies exist, which is a strong testimonial to the marketing efforts of the laxative industry. Laxatives pose a nutritional risk because they can lead to decreased absorption of certain vitamins and minerals and are more often the cause rather than the cure of gastrointestinal tract miseries.

Colon Cancer

Colon cancer rates are higher in the most economically advanced countries. In fact, this condition is almost non-existent in most traditional societies. Most theories of etiology stress a nutritional component. Identified culprits include protein (Gregor et al., 1969), sugar (Yudkin, 1972), refined carbohydrates (Cleave, 1974), excess fat (Reddy and Wynder, 1973; Drasar and Hill, 1974), and fiber depletion (Burkitt, 1971; Walker, 1974; Trowell, 1976; Walker and Burkitt, 1976).

Those researchers who stress the importance of fat in the etiology of colon cancer (Reddy and Wynder, 1973; Drasar and Hill, 1974) suggest several mechanisms of pathogenesis. It is possible that fat enhances the formation of bile acids that are then coverted into carcinogens (Hill, 1981). There is also a possibility that fat promotes tumor formation by a less clearly defined process that alters cell metabolism and tumorgenicity. In rejecting this hypothesis, Burkitt (1978) notes that cancer of the colon is four times more frequent in Demark as in Finland, even though fat consumption is the same. However, the Finns consume 80 percent more fiber than the Dames. Schaefer (1959) notes that while Eskimos have a high-fat diet, they exhibit low colon cancer rates.

High protein intake has been promoted as a possible cause of colonic cancer (Gregor et al., 1969). Visick (1975) suggests that its carcinogenic potential is related to the stimulation of increased ammonia release by cells, digestive processes, and microfloral activity. High concentration of ammonia in the bowel leads to an increase in cell formation which carries with it an increased risk of malignant cell production. Ammonia is known to alter RNA, which also may be related to increased malignant cell production.

Many researchers favor a dietary fiber hypothesis in explaining colon cancer rates. Their ideas are based on the observation that colon cancer is almost nonexistent in populations that consume significant amounts of dietary fiber. In the U.S., Seventh Day Adventists have a lower mortality rate from all malignant disease then do other Americans as well as lower rate of colon cancer. They consume a diet low in meat and fat and relatively high in fiber (Phillips, 1975).

What are the mechanisms proposed to explain the protective effect of high-fiber diets? First, it is possible that fiber acts to bind bile salts and sterols such as cholesterol. By binding bile salts fiber lessens the possibility of their conversion by bacteria to carcinogenic secondary bile acids. Fiber may also bind ingested toxins (with carcinogenic potential) and therefore promote their harmless excretion. The water binding capacity of fiber can result in increased stool weight and decreased transit time. Thus potential carcinogens can be eliminated more quickly. Increased stool volume may also serve to dilute potentially harmful substances. (Cummings, 1981).

Fiber may also alter the microflora of the gut in favor of species less likely to produce carcinogenic bile acid metabolities. Drasar and Hill (1974) noted that samples of feces from low risk populations contain less anaerobic bacteria than the feces of high risk populations. It is a possibility that fiber makes the feces more acidic, and thus less susceptible to carcinogenic activity. Howell (1975), after a study of populations in 37 countries, proposed that after diets become deficient in fiber, particular dietary components and their by-products are then able to produce cancer. She further suggests that cereals and pulses are cancer-protective.

In reviewing over 50 studies related to dietary fiber, Kelsay (1978) concluded that the evidence is not conclusive and should be interpreted with caution. Walker (1976) suggested that as a preventive measure we ought to increase our dietary intake of unrefined foods and simultaneously reduce refined carbohydrate, animal protein, and total calorie consumption. Changes in life style, such as increased physical activity (which encourages bowel motility and more rapid transit time), should be part of a preventive program. The reduction of social stress would likewise be helpful.

Carcinoma of the large bowel is the most common malignancy in those over 70 and second only to lung cancer as a killer among cancers. The incidence of colon carcinoma or rectal carcinoma increases with age, but older patients appear to have a better prognosis than younger ones (Berman and Kirsner, 1972). It is easily diagnosed with over one-half of the cases occurring within range of the examining finger and three-fourths within range of the protoscope. The five-year survival rate after surgery is 50 percent and mortality rates from surgery are quite low.

Better dietary habits in early adulthood can greatly reduce the incidence of colonic carcinoma and thus eliminate the use of surgery as a last resort. In fact, a dietary fiber change related to preventive action may be one of the simplest and easiest dietary changes to implement. The problem of colorectal cancer is one area where better nutrition education can establish eating patterns capable of preventing a major health problem for middle-aged and older Americans.

CARDIOVASCULAR DISEASE

Cardiovascular diseases including "heart attack" (myocardial infarction) and "stroke" (cerebrovascular accident) are the major causes of death and disability in the affluent world. Although such deaths appear to be declining in the United States, the American Heart Association (1978) estimates that almost 30 million Americans have some form of heart and/or blood vessel disease.

Atherosclerosis, a narrowing of the arterial passageways, is a pathological process involved in most diseases of the cardiovascular system. The exact manner in which atherosclerosis begins is not known, though the likely factors that initiate and encourage it are multiple. These include: (1) personal factors (family history, sex and age); (2) life-style factors (cigarette smoking, obesity, diet, and stress); (3) pathologic factors (the presence of other diseases such as diabetes); and (4) environmental factors (air and water pollutants, noise).

Recent research has increased the number of dietary links to cardiovascular diseases—lipid metabolism, trace element imbalances, excess sugar and refined carbohydrates, and reduced dietary fiber have received the most attention. However, the evidence supporting the involvement of the nutritional complexes is uneven and sometimes conflicting.

Early research on atherosclerosis revealed that atheroma were composed largely of lipids and consequently a great deal of investigation centered around the role of lipids in cardiovascular disease. Early work examined the role of cholesterol intake on serum cholesterol levels, and later the emphasis shifted to the role of saturated fats. More recently, the role of polyunsaturated fats in lowering cholesterol levels has been championed by clinicians and the food oil industry. The success of these efforts has been varied and not without controversy. Scientific as well as industrial critics have emerged. The elimination of certain foods as part of a cardiovascular health program is obviously not without implications for certain food industries and scientists who consult for them.

At this time, a majority of scientists favor some kind of explanation based on abnormal lipid metabolism as being important in the development of atherosclerosis. A currently popular explanation along these lines is that excessive consumption of dietary cholesterol and saturated fats along with a low intake of polyunsaturated fats results in serum lipid abnormalities. The abnormalities, such as elevated serum cholesterol, elevated low density lipoproteins, elevated triglycerides, and reduced high density lipoproteins, allow lipid accumulation in coronary arteries, which then supposedly leads to atherosclerosis. This view is not without its critics (Mann, 1977; Kannel, 1978; National Heart and Lung Institute, 1971), but the bulk of the evidence from epidemiological studies, animal studies, clinical observations, and human metabolic research seems to support the hypothesis (Krehl, 1977).

On what grounds do the critics of this diet-lipids explanation attach its validity? George Mann (1971), of the Vanderbilt University Medical School, cites evidence from the Framingham and Tecumseh studies indicating that levels of serum lipids and cholesterol were essentially unrelated to dietary practice. In addition, Mann believes that mortality trends since 1950 do not support the argument that extensive dietary modifications have had a major effect on clinical events. He also argues that no dietary therapy has been shown effective for the prevention and treatment of coronary heart disease.

Finally, according to Mann, the evidence gathered from clinical attempts to reduce cholesteremia (the presence of cholesterol in the blood) with drugs indicate little palliative effect on coronary heart disease.

Mann admits that excess cholesterol in the blood contributes to the development of heart disease and that reduction of cholesterol levels should help clinically. However, he does not associate hypercholesteremia with dietary intake of cholesterol. Rather, according to Mann (1971), something noxious in the environment such as excess vitamin D or carbon monoxide disturbs the conversion of cholesterol to bile acid and thus leads to an increase in the body's pool of cholesterol. Further, Mann finds exercise to be of greater protective value than dietary modification against the complications of atherosclerosis. Others have written of the contribution of exercise in preventing coronary heart disease (Paffenburger et al., 1977; Keys, 1980a; Morris et al., 1973).

Mann has received support from various sources (Altschule, 1978; Kannel, 1978; McMichael, 1977; Reiser, 1978), all of whom seem to be in agreement with the National Heart and Lung Institute (1917) that " . . . there is, as yet, no conclusive evidence that intervention with respect to normalizing risk factors [high cholesterol levels] will reduce the risk of atherosclerosis." Reiser (1978) suggests that rather than attempting to limit saturated fat intake for the general population those in high cholesterol levels should be identified through screening procedures and then treated.

Epidemiological studies indicate that countries, regions, and groups that are characterized by a diet low in saturated fat and cholesterol do not have significant coronary heart disease problems. However, studies such as the Ireland-Boston Heart Study (Brown et al., 1970) that compared pairs of brothers living in Boston and Ireland indicate that the type of dietary fat and cholesterol intake did not influence coronary heart disease. This investigation suggests that differences in a total complex of variables must be used to account for the fact that Bostonians have a greater risk of contracting serious athersclerotic disease than Irishmen.

Serum lipoproteins have also been implicated in the pathogenesis of coronary heart disease. Three lipoproteins are most important in this regard: (1) low density lipoprotein (LDL), very low density lipoprotein (VLDL), and high density lipoprotein (HDL), all of which function in the transport of cholesterol and other factors in the blood. VLDL and LDL allow cholesterol to become deposited on the artery walls, while HDLs seem to scavenge cholesterol and return it to the liver for excretion. Having high levels of high density lipoprotein may be a hereditary trait, but smoking, obesity, and an oversedentary life style tend to lower them. Low HDL levels appear to be dangerous and positively correlated with coronary heart disease, especially when coupled with high levels of LDL (Winick, 1980). Keys (1980b) recently reported that lower than average HDL levels was a significant predictor of death due to heart disease.

In the past, triglycerides were identified as a possible etiological factor in coronary heart disease and they received considerable attention since they appeared amenable to dietary control. More recently this attention has abated. Evidence from the Framingham Study seems to negate the significance of triglycerides in atherogenesis. Epidemiologically, many areas of the world with relatively low rates of coronary heart disease are characterized by high levels of triglycerides. Hulley and associates (1980) recently examined almost all the studies on the relationship between triglycerides and coronary heart disease. They found little support for the relationship and concluded that preventive programs should be abandoned.

A number of investigators have suggested that the increased consumption of sugar and refined carbohydrates is associated with heart disease (Yudkin, 1972; Cleave and Campbell, 1966). They note that nonwestern cultures, especially in Africa, have a lower incidence of coronary heart disease compared with the West. In addition, the absence of sugar and refined carbohydrate intake in these cultures—not fat intake—appears to be the critical factor. These studies have been criticized on both methodological and statistical grounds by Keys (1970, 1971). Further, Walker (1971) and Mann (1974) have shown that human studies on sugar and coronary heart disease have produced conflicting results.

The conflicting results may be the result of individual and synergistic factors. Some individuals may have a genetic predisposition to showing high serum lipids under the stress of high sucrose consumption. It is also possible that consumption of sugar in a high fat diet might be synergistic in the production of coronary heart disease. However, diets low in fat but high in sugar would not be expected to lead to the same results.

Dietary fiber has been suggested as being useful in the reduction of serum cholesterol. Fiber may reduce absorption of ingested cholesterol or may modify the production of endogenous cholesterol. Not all types of fiber, however, are effective in this way. For instance, pectin, rolled oats, and guar gum lower serum cholesterol while wheat fiber and cellulose do not (Kelsay, 1978; Jenkins et al., 1975).

Various trace elements have also been associated with the pathogenesis of coronary heart disease. For example, soft-water consumption is associated with a higher incidence of this disease. A number of trace-element deficiencies such as magnesium, zinc, vanadium, and calcium have also been correlated with an increased incidence of the condition.

Hypertension

Hypertension is a "silent killer" that causes 20,000 deaths annually in the United States, often striking in the prime years of life with little or no manifestation of symptoms before a major complication occurs. It is estimated that over 20 million people in the United States can be categorized as hypertensive. The condition is more prevalent in women than men, and blacks seem to be more susceptible than whites. About two-thirds of the incidence of hypertension is due to unknown causes. High blood pressure is usually its only symptom. Hypertensives have three times the rate of cardiovascular mortality as unaffected individuals. It has been suggested that genetic predisposition plays an important role in this form of hypertension, and nutrition, especially sodium intake, also seems to be a contributing factor. In fact, sodium may be an environmental stimulus that leads to the development of hypertension in genetically susceptible people.

Animal studies have produced hypertension in rats by adding salt to their regular diet. However, it appears that rats who are exposed to high salt intake from youth develop higher blood pressures than old rats that are first exposed to high levels later in life. Dahl (1972) suggests that sodium intake in early childhood may be a significant factor in the development of hypertension in adulthood. Further, he studied five population groups with a lifetime salt intake of four to 25 grams per day, and noted a positive correlation between high salt intake and the presence of hypertension. The Framingham project and other studies have not found a positive correlation between salt intake and hypertension. Dahl and his associates (1972) suggest that some individuals are more or less resistant to the detrimental effects of salt, and that development of hypertension under the stimulus of salt is related to this differentiation.

Excessive body weight and/or body fat has long been associated with hypertension, and most programs of hypertensive control include weight loss. Some researchers believe that unless an individual is grossly obese, there is little effect on blood pressure. Lauer and his team (1976) argue that whether high blood pressure and high body weight are positively correlated cannot be determined at this time, although they do suggest that weight may account for about 10 percent of the blood pressure variation in a population. However, many obese people do not have high blood pressure.

It has been estimated that one to three grams a day of dietary sodium is sufficient to replace sodium lost by excretion, although individuals with some forms of kidney disease may require more. The average North American intake is six to 18 grams a day. The recently established and still controversial U. S. Dietary Goals recommend five grams daily as a preventive measure for hypertension. Lowering sodium intake in the United States would be a difficult task, since great amounts of highly processed and fast food used in this country are often high in sodium content. Artificial sources of sodium include sodium bicarbonate (baking soda and powder), sodium phosphate (some cheese and cereal), sodium alginate (ice cream and chocolate drink), sodium sulfate (fruit preservative), and sodium saccharine (low calorie sweetener), among others. Natural foods high in sodium include milk, meat, cheese, eggs, poultry, fish, beets, carrots, celery, kale, and spinach.

Use of sodium restriction (1500–2000 mg./day) has been advocated as a replacement for drugs in the treatment of hypertension (Morgan et al., 1978).

This has not gone unchallenged, though clinical evidence does seem to indicate that moderate sodium restriction can lower blood pressure and thus prevent at least mild hypertension (Albanese, 1980). Most practitioners who use this approach today prefer reduction of sodium intake to one gram a day plus the use of a diuretic.

ENDOCRINE DISORDERS: DIABETES MELLITUS

Diabetes is an ancient disease. It was first described in the Egyptian Ebeas papyrus in 1500 B.C. It is a true disease of civilization—prevalence rates increase with urbanization, sedentary life styles, modern work patterns, and the dietary changes associated with modern life. As early as diabetes was recognized, it was not until 1788 that Rollo proposed a sound dietary approach to the treatment of diabetes.

Diabetes is the fifth most prominent cause of disease-related death in the United States. It is estimated that over 10 million people in the United States are affected by diabetes, and its prevalence appears to be increasing at an annual rate of 6 percent. A 1977 estimate by the U.S. Department of Health, Education and Welfare suggests that this condition costs about six billion dollars annually in the form of medical expenses and lost productivity. In terms of individual affliction, diabetes can lead to blindness, kidney failure, stroke, and gangrene in the extremities. Coronary heart disease, due to blood vessel degeneration, is twice as likely in victims of diabetes than in their unafflicted counterparts.

As a result of increasing life expectancy and effective management of the disease, diabetics generally live long lives. In fact, there is a growing number of older diabetics. Besides those who have had the disease since youth, older diabetics include those who have developed it in late middle age and those who first manifest if in later life. The latter group often experience the mildest course of pathology and are easier to manage.

However, many cases of diabetes go unnoticed, so the exact incidence among the elderly is unknown, though there appears to be a steady increase in its incidence from childhood to old age. The rate peaks between the ages of 65 to 75 at 64.4/1000 tested, and at 75 drops to 57.9/1000 people tested. It is estimated that 20 percent of all diabetics are 60 years or over and that 5 percent of the entire population over 65 are diabetic (USPHS, 1978).

Diabetes is not a single disease entity, and at least two general categories of the condition are recognized. Type I is known as idiopathic insulin-dependent diabetes (or juvenile diabetes), while Type II is called idiopathic insulin-independent diabetes (adult onset). There is little evidence to suggest a nutritional component in the etiology of Type I, which is probably associated with an immunulogical disturbance possibly influenced by heredity or a viral infection. Type II, the most common kind of diabetes, is associated with obesity and possibly enkephalin sensitivity (Baird, 1980).

Diabetes is easily missed in the elderly because of several factors. First, the classical symptoms of thirst, increased urination, severe wasting or weakness, and elevated fasting levels of blood glucose are rarely present. Second, hyperglycemia can occur without glycosuria, and finally, the condition's symptoms may be confused with those of other conditions common among the elderly, such as congestive heart failure, uremia, and cholecystitis. It should also be noted that overdiagnosis of diabetes occurs in some cases. This may occur if the diagostician uses only the standard tests. For instance, glucose tolerance normally decreases with age, thus affecting norm interpretations. There is also much disagreement on the kinds of diagnostic criteria that can be efficaciously applied to older persons.

The mortality rates for those who are over 60 and diabetic are higher than for the general population (Kart et al., 1978). The long-term complications of diabetes are numerous and must be considered when planning for its management. For example, vascular disease is responsible for about 75 percent of the deaths from diabetes. Atherosclerosis progresses twice as fast in diabetics, and coronary heart disease is twice as common in diabetic men and five times as common in diabetic women than in the general population.

A simple cause and effect relationship between diet and diabetes does not exist, but the American Diabetes Association (1974) suggests that improved nutrition could reduce its incidence in the United States by 30 percent. Most researchers would probably agree that obesity is the one proven diabetogenic factor. In fact, some researchers believe that diabetes is the only significant pathological condition related to being overweight (Mann, 1971). Diabetes is rare in societies where obesity is uncommon. In the U.S., approximately 75 percent of those with adult onset diabetes are obese, and obese people are three times more likely to manifest diabetes than those of normal weight.

Baird (1980) found that in all social classes and in both sexes that the incidence of obesity was higher among diabetics. Further, she could not find any significant difference in either the quality of food consumed by her general samples of obese and nonobese subjects. However, those with diabetes ate significantly more food than nondiabetics. It also is significant that weight loss does reverse some of the metabolic disturbances of diabetes. In an early piece of research, Newburgh and Conn (1939) showed that weight loss corrected abnormal glucose tolerance in 90 percent of a middle aged population.

The search for qualitative nutritional factors that promote diabetogenesis is very controversial and plagued with contradictory results. Nutritional factors could be involved relative to damage to the pancreas, impaired glucose tolerance, and impaired function of the beta cells. Little experimental data is available to strongly support a nutritional basis for any of these mechanisms.

Epidemiological studies correlating diabetes with dietary variations are abundant, but the evidence presented is generally inconclusive. Himsworth (1949), noting the fall in diabetic mortality during wartime, proposed that a high fat diet was diabetogenic since fat consumption noticeably dropped during wartime food shortages. However, he failed to consider that sucrose consumption also dropped abruptly and significantly at this time. Other data available at the time would also have pointed out that Eskimos have a diet very high in animal fat, but still exhibit a very low incidence of diabetes.

A number of researchers have sought a correlation between a high incidence of diabetes and consumption of sucrose, or refined sugar. Cohen (1961) noted that Yemenite Jews emigrating to Israel had a low incidence of diabetes. However, after a period of years in Israel and adoption of a typical Israeli diet that included 20 to 25 percent of the total calories coming from sucrose, prevalence rates increased to approximately those of western countries. Campbell (1963) arrived at conclusions similar to Cohen's while studying Asians and Africans in and around Durban in South Africa. Cleave and Campbell (1966) also found diabetes related to the increased use of refined sugar in the Natal area of India. Yudkin (1969) demonstrated a significant correlation between the amount of sugar consumed and mortality from diabetes in 22 countries.

A number of other epidemiologists found little data in their studies to support a sucrose-diabetes relationship. Baird (1972), in Scotland, found no relationship between sugar consumption and diabetes, while similar studies in England came to the same conclusion. Poon-King and associates (1968) studied five geographical districts in Trinidad and found the incidence of diabetes lowest in districts with highest per capita consumption of sugar. In the South Pacific, Prior (1974) found variations in diabetes not accounted for by dietary consumption of sugar and suggested that other environmental factors as yet unidentified might be more important. Is it possible that some individuals, or even populations, may have a genetically based sensitivity to sucrose? If so, it might be possible to prevent diabetes in such populations by having them avoid high-sucrose stimulation. (Cleave and Campbell 1966).

Trowell (1975) and others have suggested a link between fiber-depleted diets and a high incidence of diabetes. He noted that mortality from diabetes fell in Britain during the world wars when a coarser, less refined flour was consumed. The same researcher (Trowell, 1978) suggested that the incorporation of fiber into the diet may lower blood insulin and blood glucose levels. Miranda and Horowitz (1978) support this contention. The specific effects of selected components of the dietary fiber complex are also being investigated in relation to lowering the incidence of diabetes. It must be remembered that when dietary fiber is increased, the protein, fat, vitamin and/or mineral content of the diet may be altered as well, and these factors must be considered in any explanation of observed effects.

Mild, late-onset diabetes can often be controlled by dietary restrictions of carbohydrates of around 100 grams a day. Although the amount of complex carbohydrates allowed can be quite variable, 30 to 40 percent of the total calorie intake in complex carbohydrates seems reasonable initially. Occasionally a diet that is 65 percent complex carbohydrates can be tolerated. Sucrose and sucrose-containing foods, as well as glucose, lactose, and fructose additives should be excluded.

In the past, two methods were used in the care of older diabetics. One stressed strict and rigorous diet control while the other allowed more freedom in selecting a diet and used insulin to control hypoglycemia. In the late 1950s the introduction of the oral hypoglycemic tablet led to the neglect of dietary therapy and promoted an overdependence on medication. The negative impact of this abuse has yet to be determined.

A balanced diet is the key to the management of diabetes. It is important to keep in mind that the lifelong food habits of an individual will be difficult to change. Recent dietary recommendations suggest lower amounts of fat, saturated fat, and cholesterol, and higher amounts of complex carbohydrates than are typical of the north American diet. Of course, the less a diet is manipulated and modified to achieve balance, the greater the probability of adherence to the diet. A number of principles in dietary management of diabetes are important:

1. A diet should be compatible with an individual's economic and social background.

2. A diet should be compatiable with an individual's activity profile (exercise helps weight control).

3. A diet should be made up of readily available, commonly used foods.

4. A diet should plan three well-balanced, regularly-spaced meals with small, nutritious snacks in between (especially for those taking insulin).

5. Foods high in pure sugar must be eliminated.

6. A diet should contain a balance of carbohydrate, protein, and fat at the following approximate levels: 45 to 55 percent carbohydrate, 10 to 20 percent protein, and 30 to 35 percent fat.

7. Adequate salt intake must be assured, and potassium should be watched; chromium supplements might be helpful to those who do not respond well to insulin.

8. A broad-spectrum multivitamin supplement might be helpful, since excretion of water-soluble vitamins is often excessive.

OBESITY AND WEIGHT CONTROL AMONG THE ELDERLY

Determining whether an individual is overweight or obese is more difficult than it would seem. By one definition, obesity is present when the accumulation of fat in body tissue is equal to or more than 20 percent of the body weight in males and 30 percent in females. However, one can be overweight without being fat, with the excess weight being muscle, as is seen for example, in football players and weightlifters.

Diagnosing obesity poses at least as many problems as defining it. Appearance is oftened used, but does not differentiate between fat, muscle, and water accumulation. Weight and height tables are difficult to use with the elderly because of their lessened physical stature. These tables have recently come under criticism for persons of all ages since, even when body build is controlled for, they tend to underestimate ideal weight by as much as 20 percent. X-rays are hazardous and expensive and flotation techniques are impractical for most people. An accurate approach in the determination of obesity involves the use of skinfold measurements, although the elderly present special problems for this technique due to age-related skin changes. Triceps skinfold thickness is a measure of subcutaneous fat and is considered an index of the body's energy stores. Precision in measurement is absolutely necessary. In addition, as with weight in general, measurements must be evaluated in terms of actual age, height, and even the theoretically correct weight for a given age.

Estimates of obesity in the general American population vary between 25 and 45 percent. Data on older adults is available from the Ten-State Nutrition Survey (See Chapter Three). Older black women had the highest prevalence of obesity—over 45 percent in the 45 to 60 year-old group. More than one-third of all white women aged 55 to 65 years in the survey were defined as obese. Among the elderly, the lowest prevalence of obesity was found in black males. The HANES data show a similar pattern. In both studies, low income was associated with a higher prevalence of obesity.

Some obesity is juvenile in its onset. Overeating in childhood may give rise to fat tissue containing large numbers of fat cells. One hypothesis is that an excess of fat cells makes it difficult to keep weight off because these cells have to be depleted before a normal weight can be reached. However, a number of researchers have challenged the methodological basis of this hypothesis (Salans, et al., 1973).

Another form of obesity is called adult onset and appears in the middle years of adulthood. This obesity usually has its origin in overeating, ignorance of proper nutrition, and reduced activity. Metabolic problems probably account for only small fraction (perhaps 2 percent) of all obesity in aulthood.

The hazards of obesity for people of all ages are reported as adversely affecting almost every system of the body (Price and Pritts, 1980). Life expectancy is lower and morbidity rates are higher. High blood pressure, gall bladder problems, coronary heart disease, diabetes, and postsurgical complications are more prevalent among the obese. However, Mann (1971) is not sure that obesity by itself is bad. Becoming obese through diminished activity and increased consumption of refined sugar and fats is another matter. He states that the effect of obesity alone as predictor of heart disease is very small and of borderline statistical significance. Recent research by Keys (1980a, b) also tends to support a less negative approach to the effects of being overweight.

estimates that basic metabolism declines 16 percent between 20 and 70 years of age, necessitating a decrease in caloric intake of approximately one-third. Ahrens (1970) calculated a per decade decline of 43 calories/day in the requirements for males from age 25 on and a per decade decline of 27 calories/day for females from age 25 on. It is likely that this change is due to alterations in basal metabolism, body composition, and activities related to aging per se. In addition to basic metabolic decline, many of the elderly are subject to additional stresses that contribute to obesity. These include grief, economic insecurity, and social isolation, to name a few. In such cases, socio-psychological counseling, support, and contact with others may be more important in dealing with the problem of obesity than nutrition education or medical aid. Advertising encourages eating in general and heavily emphasizes sugar and snack foods that can contribute to caloric imbalance. Affluence allows us to eat for entertainment and pleasure rather than for subsistence. At the same time, we can afford labor-saving devices that save human energy. Modern processing allows us to eat low bulk foods that are sweet and highly refined simply for their great palatability. Paradoxically, impoverished people may become obese because cost forces them to eat high calorie foods that are generally cheaper than protective foods.

What available weight control methods are functional for the elderly? Logically, reduced intake of food along with increased activity go a long way in controlling weight. The elderly (like everybody else) must be educated to moderation in these matters. Realistic goals should be established, meals should not be skipped, and plateaus in weight loss must be anticipated. It is also wise to avoid eating out, since little control over food preparation can be exerted and the social atmosphere is conducive to overeating. A reduction of about 500 calories a day can result in the loss of one pound a week. Some people have found a pattern of one day on diet and one day off to be successful, especially for weight maintenance.

Crash diets, including fasting and novelty diets, can be harmful and should be avoided. Real medical problems may be aggravated or potentiated by such diets. Dietary regulation with drugs should be approached with caution and medical supervision. Even under supervision, the usefulness of so-called "diet pills" is limited, and tolerance can develop, necessitating an increased dosage. Initial success in weight loss is often nullified by a "rebound effect," which finds the individual eating more than before to compensate for feelings of deprivation.

In the elderly, drugs present special problems for weight loss because of interaction with other medications and potential errors of dose and timing. Liquid protein formulations designed for the extremely obese (50 pounds overweight) should probably be avoided. Though reactions vary individually, these formulas can be extremely dangerous. Over 40 deaths, most often related to calcium and potassium imbalances, have been associated with their use (Lantigua et al., 1980).

Increased activity, even exercise, should be a part of any dietary plan, though age and the existence of chronic disease or disability must be taken into account. Strenuous activity can decrease appetite, raise resting metabolism, and increase muscular efficiency and tone. The psychological lift, sense of achievement, improved self-image, and confidence many of the elderly get from participation in activity and exercise programs cannot be overlooked. Positive aspects of exercise carry over into daily activities related to psychosocial well being, eating habits, and overall health maintenance.

ALCOHOLISM

Estimates of the alcoholic population in the U.S. range from nine to ten million adults. How many of these are elderly is unknown. In general, the elderly seem to exhibit a lower incidence of alcoholism than do younger groups, although as a result of their "invisibility," much of the alcoholism among the aged may go unnoticed.

Alcoholism in old age is of two types: lifelong and late-life. Lifelong alcoholism formerly was associated with cirrhosis of the liver (ninth leading killer in the U.S.) and early death. However, due to modern medical technology, the use of antibiotics, better nutritional therapy, and advanced hospital treatment, many alcoholics survive well into old age. Late-life alcoholism may be the result of grief, depression, loneliness, boredom, and/or chronic pain. Alcohol can become a tool for coping with many of the stresses of old age.

Alcohol is a common contributor to malnourishment among adults in the U.S. because of the numerous ways it interferes physiologically with nutritional status: (1) it is often used as a replacement for essential nutrients in the diet; (2) it diminishes appetite; (3) it causes inflammation of the gastrointestinal tract leading to malabsorption; and (4) it alters metabolism in such a way as to change nutrient requirements or the pathways of nutrient utilization. According to Iber (1971), 20,000 alcoholics a year suffer from nutritional conditions that necessitate hospitalization.

In heavy drinkers, alcohol may furnish up to 50 percent of the total intake of calories. These calories are "empty," contributing little else to the diet but energy. However, even though alcohol liberates 7.1 calories per gram, its food value may be less than that of an isocaloric equivalent of carbohydrate (Winick, 1981). Piorola and Lieber (1972) report that wasteful metabolic mechanisms result in alcohol calories not being fully utilized. The exact mechanisms are still unclear, but Winick (1981) suggests that they may have a relationship to increased metabolic rates and cites the observation that increased oxygen consumption accompanies the ingestion of ethanol, or alcohol, even in non-alcoholics. It is therefore possible to lose weight by the substitution of equivalent caloric units of ethanol for carbohydrates.

Malnutrition in alcoholics may be related to a number of factors other than nutrient displacement. Diminished appetite, for example, is common in alcoholics. This condition may also be due to psychological stress, the possible appetite suppressant qualities of alcohol, and neurological disorders that affect daily functioning. Alcohol can cause an inflammation of the stomach, pancreas, and intestines, thus interfering with normal digestion and possibly leading to malnutrition and impaired absorption of fat, folate, thiamine, and vitamin B_{12} in alcoholics. It is also probable that due to the dynamic interrelationship of nutrients, an increase in alcohol consumption increases the physiological requirement for nutrients such as thiamine that are involved in alcohol metabolism. In addition, the utilization of some vitamins including pyridoxine, folate, and thiamine may be impaired through deactivation and other mechanisms.

A number of the detrimental nutritional effects of alcoholism result from related liver damage. Alcohol has a direct toxic effect on the liver, which leads to hepatitis, fatty infiltration, and cirrhosis. In the absence of normal liver function, lipid metabolism becomes abnormal, causing increased concentrations of triglycerides and all of the lipoprotein factions. Further, the hepatic stores of folate B_6, B_{12}, and niacin may be subject to depletion. Abnormal vitamin D activation in combination with alcohol intake and defectively low intestinal absorption could contribute to the increased incidence of fractures observed in alcoholics (Korsten and Lieber, 1979). The liver is also important in the production of bile salts necessary in fat digestion as well as in the synthesis of clotting factors. Roe (1981) reports that alcohol can damage the precursor blood cells of the bone marrow, thus increasing the need for blood-forming nutrients such as folacin, B_6, and B_{12}.

In the elderly, the above risks can be complicated by age-related changes in the body's digestive, absorptive, and assimilative capacities. For example, alcohol-related changes in absorptive capacity can be coupled with an age-associated decline in the nourishing capacity of blood vessels (Kart, Metress, Metress, 1978). For elderly people on nutrionally marginal diets, excess alcohol consumption can lead to a state of overt malnutrition due to such physiological changes.

CANCER AND DIET

Current understanding of the role of diet in the etiology of cancer is largely based on epidemiological surveys, though case control studies in humans and experimental data from animal studies are supportive of the diet-cancer connection. This epidemiological research suggests that environmental factors are important in the production or origin of cancer. Cancer incidence varies widely geographically, and its incidence has a tendency to change when people move from low-risk to high-risk areas. Some epidemiological evidence suggests that diet may be correlated with more than half the cancers in women and at least one-third of all cancers in men (Gori, 1981; Wynder and Gori, 1977). Especially susceptible sites are the breast, colon, and stomach. Many of these cancers often manifest themselves in later years, although their pathogenesis may have begun during middle age or earlier. The most thoroughly studied diet-cancer relationships are related to colon cancer incidence (discussed above).

Oace (1978) suggests three mechanisms that may be involved in diet-related carcinogenesis. First, ingested food might contain carcinogens in the form of additives or natural toxic substances. Second, some foods contain compounds that can be converted during processing, cooking, and digestion to carcinogens—for example nitrosamines that originate from nitrite additives. Finally, the balance of micronutrients such as fat, carbohydrate, protein, and dietary fiber may influence the development of cancer through changes in gastrointestinal tract ecology or by making cells more susceptible to malignant changes.

Correlations have been reported between cancer and high poly-unsaturated fat (PUFA) intake. Pearse and Dayton (1971) note that the incidence of fatal carcinoma is high in people with four times the normal intake of PUFA and half as much cholesterol as normal. While Rose and associates (1974) suggest that high PUFA could stimulate bile soft formations, a necessary substrate for carcinogenic bacteria, Mertin (1973) proposes that PUFA inhibits the immune system, and, therefore, aberrant cells that normally would be removed from circulation remain active.

Correlations have also been reported between high-fat intake and the incidence of breast cancer. The mechanism is unclear, but it may be related to anaerobic bacteria that produce estrogen from biliary steroids or elevation of serum prolactin that acts to promote tumorgenesis (Brammer and DeFelice, 1980).

Anticarcinogens are substances that directly or indirectly prevent the production of cancer. They may accomplish this by direct antagonism or by interfering with the activation of carcinogens. Vitamin A may act as an anti-carcinogen by changing the sensitivity of tissues or by altering essential metabolites (Sporn and Newton, 1979). Graham (1980) cites a number of studies that hint of a protective role for vitamin A. However, Peto (1981) suggests that the provitamin beta-carotene, not retinal, reduces the incidence of cancer in man. This relationship was confirmed in relation to lung cancer risk by the research of Shekelle and associates (1981). Cameron and colleagues (1979) suggest that vitamin C availability may be related to resistance to cancer, especially as an inhibitor of nitrosamine formation. The antioxidants and BHT and BHA have exhibited some anticarcinogenesis while selenium and zinc salts also exhibit similar potential.

Graham (1980) cites a study by Bjelke that noted a lower risk of colon cancer among individuals eating large amounts of cruciferous vegetables such as cabbage, broccoli and brussel sprouts. It is possible that they may protect against tumor production through indoles that help in the detoxification of carcinogens.

Young and Newberne (1981), after reviewing the relationship between vitamins and the prevention of cancer, suggest caution in such speculation. They contend that no evidence supports recommending major changes in vitamin intake as a preventive measure against cancer. In addition, they disavow any use of vitamin megadoses. However, Newberne (1978) indicates that it is critical to learn more about how dietary factors affect carcinogenesis in order to use such information in the prevention of cancer. After a considerable review of the evidence, Reddy and associates (1980) recommend the following dietary steps to prevent cancer: 1) reduce fat consumption from 40 to 20 percent, 2) increase dietary bulk from cereal brans, vegetables and fruit fiber, 3) ensure adequate amounts of vitamins A and C, the trace elements zinc and selenium, and, less importantly, vitamin E and riboflavin.

Seventh Day Adventists pursue a lacto-ovo-vegetarian diet that is characterized by 25 percent less fat and 50 percent more fiber than the average nonvegetarian diet. At the same time, the proportion of saturated fat is doubled (Phillips, 1975). Cancer mortality statistics indicate that Adventists have cancer rates (unrelated to smoking and drinking) from most sites that are 50 to 70 percent that of the general population. In addition to low fat and high fiber consumption, the Adventist diet includes fewer calories, relatively low protein intake, high intake of vitamins A and C and abstinence from coffee, tea, and alcohol.

Bill (1975) suggests that the typical Adventist diet might influence the functioning of the immune system. Adventists show a reduced incidence of cancer in all sites, suggesting a stronger "defense" system. It is possible that low intake of foreign animal protein increases the ability of the immune system to recognize and destroy the cancerous cells before they are able to realize their destructive potential.

The idea that nutritional status may play an important part in carcinogenesis has become widespread and is deserving of attention. Further, the impact of dietary factors on the prevention of tumor production must also be investigated. This research is necessary not only for application in preventive medicine, but to combat pseudoscientific treatment regimens based on insufficient or erroneous evidence. Cancer prevention is a field susceptible to quackery and deceit. The notion that cancer means certain death is still widespread and creates anxiety among those who have the disease as well as those close to them. They may be quite receptive to simplistic remedies that may be expensive, ineffective, and, in some cases, dangerous.

SUMMARY

Scientists do not always agree on the involvement of nutrition in disease etiology. Some of this disagreement is methodological in nature. Much of the evidence on the relationship between nutrition and aging and disease is epidemiological. These kinds of studies are often not supported by experimental data.

Disease and disability conditions that have a nutritional component are not exclusive to older adulthood, though a significant proportion of older adults are affected by them. Nutritional status can interact with normal biological aging or with pathological aging processes. The diseases and disability conditions reviewed in this chapter are decubitus ulcers, osteoporosis, osteomalacia, osteoarthritis, rheumatoid arthritis, gout, Parkinson's disease, dental caries, periodontal disease, hiatus hernia, gall stones, liver disease, diverticulosis, hemorrhoids, constipation, cardiovascular disease including hypertension, diabetes mellitus, obesity, alcoholism, and cancer.

STUDY QUESTIONS

1. Why is there disagreement over the nature and significance of various nutritional factors in the etiology of disease?
2. Discuss osteoporosis and its significance for the health of the elderly. Identify and discuss some of the major factors possibly involved in the development of osteoporosis.
3. Differentiate between osteomalacia and osteoporosis. Identify the possible dietary components involved in the development of each.
4. What is the role of nutrition in the development of:
   a. osteoarthritis;
   b. rheumatoid arthritis;
   b. gout?
5. What are the three major factors necessary for the development of dental caries? What role do sucrose, saliva, protein, fats, and phosphates play in tooth decay? How important is fluorine in caries prevention?
6. What are the major factors related to the development of periodontal disease? How is nutrition involved? What is the relationship between periodontal disease and osteoporosis?
7. Identify the possible nutritional components and/or implications in the following disorders:
   a. hiatus hernia;
   b. cholelithiasis;
   c. liver disease;
   d. diverticulosis;
   e. hemorrhoids;
   f. constipation.
8. Discuss the possible relationship between diet and colon cancer. What are the mechanisms proposed to explain the protective effect of a high fiber diet?
9. Identify atherosclerosis and the major factors that initiate and en-

courage its development. What is the role of lipids in cardiovascular disease? On what grounds do critics attack the diet-lipid hypothesis? What role do lipoproteins, triglycerides, dietary fiber, and sucrose consumption play in the development of atherosclerosis?

10. Discuss the relationship between salt and hypertension. Why is it so difficult to reduce sodium intake in the United States?

11. Identify diabetes. What are the implications of the following for diabetes: obesity, sucrose consumption, fat consumption, dietary fiber? What are some of the major principles involved in the treatment of diabetes?

12. Why is an accurate diagnosis of obesity so difficult? Distinguish between juvenile and adult-onset obesity. Why does Mann disagree with the idea that obesity in itself is bad?

13. Is obesity a special problem for the elderly? List some important principles of weight control for the elderly.

14. Identify the two types of alcoholism associated with old age. In what ways does alcoholism contribute to malnourishment? What are the special risks associated with alcoholism in the elderly?

15. What are the mechanisms that are probably involved in diet-related carcinogenesis? What steps may be of aid in the dietary prevention of cancer? In what ways are the dietary studies of Seventh Day Adventists significant for studies of the diet-cancer relationship?

BIBLIOGRAPHY

AHRENS, R. A., *Nutrition For Health.* Belmont, California: Wadsworth, 1970.

ALBANESE, A. A., "Calcium Nutrition in the Elderly," *Postgraduate Medicine*, 63, No. 3 (1976), 167–172.

_____., "Calcium Nutrition in the Elderly," *Nutrition and the M.D.*, 5 (12) (1979), 1–2.

_____., *Nutrition for the Elderly.* New York: Alan R. Liss, 1980.

_____, et al., "Problems of Bone Health in the Elderly: A Ten Year Study," *New York State Journal of Medicine*, 75 (1975), 326–336.

ALFANO, M. C., "Controversies, Perspectives and Clinical Implications of Nutrition in Periodontal Disease," *Dental Clinics of North America*, 20 (3) (1976), 519–548.

ALTSHULE, M. D., *Nutritional Factors in General Medicine: Effects of Stress and Distorted Diets.* Springfield, Illinois: C. C. Thomas, 1978.

American Diabetes Association. *Annual Report - 1974.* ADA, New York, 1974.

American Heart Association, *Heart Facts.* Dallas: American Heart Association, 1978.

AVIOLI, L. V., "The Osteoporosis Problem," in *Nutritional Disorders of American Women*, M. Winick, ed. New York: John Wiley, 1977.

BAHN, A. N., "Microbial Potential in the Etiology of Periodontal Disease," *Journal of Periodontology*, 41 (1970), 603–610.

BAIRD, J. D., "Diet and the Development of Clinical Diabetes," *Acta Latina*, 9 (1972), 621–637.

_____, "Diet and the Development of Clinical Diabetes in Man," *Proceeding of the Nutritional Society*, 40 (1981), 213-217.

BARZEL, U., *Osteoporosis*. New York: Grune and Stratton, 1970.

BERMAN, P. M. and J. B. KIRSNER, "The Aging Gut: Diseases of the Esophagus, Small Intestine and Appendix," *Geriatrics*, 27 (1972), 84-89.

BERMAN, P. M. and J. B. KIRSNER, "The Aging Gut II: Diseases of the Colon, Pancreas, Liver, and Gall Bladder, Functional Bowl Disease and Iatrogenic Disease," *Geriatrics*, 27 (1972), 117-124.

BERNSTEIN, D. S. et al., "Prevalence of Osteoporosis in High and Low Fluoride Areas in North Dakota," *Journal of American Medical Association*, 198 (1966), 85-87.

BERTOLINI, A. M. *Gerontologic Metabolism*. Springfield, Illinois: C.C. Thomas, 1969.

BILL, D. M., "Nutrition and Tumor Immunity: Divergent Effects of Anti-Tumor Antibody," *Cancer Research*, 35 (1975), 3317-3319.

BOLLET, A., et al., "Epidemiology of Osteoporosis," *Archives of Internal Medicine* 116 (1965), 191-194.

BRAMMER, S. and R. L. DeFELICE, "Dietary Advice in Regard to Risk for Colon and Breast Cancer," *Preventive Medicine*, 9 (1980), 544-549.

BRICK, I. B. and H. I. AMORY, "Incidence of Hiatus Hernia in Patients Without Symptoms," *Archives of Surgery*, 60 (1950), 1045.

BROWN, J. et al., "Nutritional and Epidemiologic Factors Related to Heart Disease," *World Review Nutrition and Dietetics*, 12 (1970), 1-42.

BULLAMORE, J. R., et al., "Effect of Age on Calcium Absorption," *Lancet*, 2 (1970), 535-537.

BURKITT, D. P., "Etiology of Cancer of the Colon and Rectum," *Cancer*, 18 (1971), 3-13.

_____ "The Link Between Low-Fiber Diets and Disease," *Human Nature*, 1 (1978), 34-41.

BUSSE, E. W., "How Mind, Body and Environment Influence Nutrition in the Elderly," *Postgraduate Medicine*, 63 (1978), 118-125.

CAMERON, E., et al., "Ascorbic Acid and Cancer: A Review," *Cancer Research*, 39 (1979), 663-681.

CAMPBELL, G. D., "Diabetes in Asians and Africans in and around Durban," *South African Medical Journal*, 37 (1963), 1195-1208.

CHALMERS, J., et al., "Osteomalacia—A Common Disease in the Elderly Woman," *Journal of Bone and Joint Surgery*, 49, No. 3 (1967), 403-423.

CLEAVE, T. L., *The Saccharine Disease*, Bristol: Wright and Sons, 1974.

_____ and C. D. CAMPBELL, *Diabetes, Coronary Thrombosis and the Saccharine Disease*. Bristol: J. D. Wright, 1966.

COHEN, A. M., "Prevalence of Diabetes Among Different Ethnic Jewish Groups," *Metabolism*, 10 (1961), 50-58.

CONNELL, A. M.., et al., Variation of Bowel Habits in Two Population Samples," *British Medical Journal*, 5470 (1965), 1095-1099.

CUMMINGS, J. H., "Dietary Fibre and Large Bowel Cancer," *Proceedings of the Nutrition Society*, 40 (1981), 7-14.

DAHL, L. K., et al., "Salt and Hypertension," *American Journal of Clinical Nutrition*, 25 (1972), 231-244.

DEPOALA, D. P. and M. C. ALFANO, "Diet and Oral Health," *Nutrition Today*, 12 No. 3 (1977), 6-11.

DRASAR, B. S. and H. J. HILL, *Human Intestinal Flora*. New York: Academic Press, 1974.

ELLIS, F. R., et al., "Incidence of Osteoporosis in Vegetarians and Omnivores," *American Journal of Clinical Nutrition*, 25 (1972), 555-558.

GALLAGHER, J. C., "Intestinal Calcium Absorption and Serum Vitamin D Metabolites in Normal Subjects and Osteoporotic Patients Effect of Age and Dietary Calcium," *Journal of Clinical Investigation*, 64 (1979), 729-736.

GARN, S. M., "Bone Loss and Aging," in *The Physiology and Pathology of Human Aging*, Ed. by R. Goldman and M. Rockstein. New York: Academic Press, 1975.

GLASS, R. L., et al., "Prevalence of Human Dental Caries and Water Borne Trace Metals," *Archives of Oral Biology*, 18 (1973), 1099-1104.

GORI, G. B., "The Cancer and Other Connections . . . if Any," *Nutrition Today*, 16 (1981), 14-22.

GRAHAM, S., "Diet and Cancer," *American Journal of Epidemiology*, 112 (1980), 2:247-252.

GREGOR, O., et al., "Gastrointestinal Cancer and Nutrition," *Gut*, 10 (1969), 1031-1034.

HILL, M. J., "Dietary Fat and Human Cancer," *Proceedings of the Nutrition Society*, 40 (1981), 15-19.

HIMSWORTH, H. P., "The Syndrome of Diabetes and Its Causes," *Lancet* 1, (1949), 465-472.

HOWELL, M. A., "Diet as an Etiological Factor in the Development of Cancers of the Colon and Rectum," *Journal of Chronic Disease*, 28 (1975), 67-80.

HULLEY, S. B., et al., "Epidemiology as a Guide to Clinical Decisions: The Association Between Triglyceride and Coronary Heart Disease," *New England Journal of Medicine*, 302 (1980), 1383-1389.

IBER, F. L., "In Alcoholism the Liver Sets the Pace," *Nutrition Today*, 6 (1971), 2-9.

JENKINS, D. J., et al., "Effects of Pectin, Guar Gum and Wheat Fiber on Serum Cholesterol. *Lancet*, 1 (1975), 116.

JOWSEY, J., et al., "Long Term Experience with Fluoride and Fluoride Combination Treatment of Osteoporosis," in *Calcium Metabolism, Bone, and Metabolic Diseases*, Ed. by F. Kuhlencordt and H. P. Kruse. New York: Springer-Verlag, 1975.

————, "Osteoporosis: Its Nature and the Role of Diet," *Post Graduate Medicine*, 60 No. 2, (1976), 75-79.

————, "Osteoporosis: Dealing with a Crippling Bone Disease of the Elderly," *Geriatrics*, 32 (1977), 41-50.

KANNEL, W. B., "Status of Coronary Heart Disease Risk Factors," *Journal of Nutrition Education*, 10, No. 1 (1978), 10-14.

KART, C., E. METRESS, and S. METRESS, *Aging and Health*. Menlo Park, California: Addison-Wesley, 1978.

KELSAY, J. L., "A Review of Research on Effects of Fiber Intake in Man," *American Journal of Clinical Nutrition*, 31 (1978), 1:142-159.

KEYS, A., "Coronary Heart Disease in Seven Countries, *Circulation*, 41 (Supplement 1) (1970), 1-211.

————, "Sucrose in the Diet and Coronary Heart Disease," *Atherosclerosis*, 14 (1971), 193-202.

————, "Overweight, Obesity, Coronary Heart Disease and Mortality," *Nutrition Today*, 15, (4) (1980a), 16-22.

————, "Alpha Lipoprotein," *Lancet* 2, (1980b), 603-606.

KIM, Y. and H. M. LINKSWEILER, "Effect of Level of Protein Intake on Calcium Metabolism and Renal Function in the Adult Human Male," *Journal of Nutrition*, 109 (1979), 1399-1404.

KORSTEN, M. A. and C. S. LIEBER, "Nutrition in the Alcoholic," *Medical Clinics of North America*, 63 (1979), 963.

KREHL, W. A., "The Nutritional Epidemiology of Cardiovascular Disease," in *Food and Nutrition in Health and Disease*, Ed. by N. H. Ross and J. Mayer. New York Academy of Science, 1977.

LAFLAMME, G. H. and J. JOWSEY, "Bone and Soft-Tissue Changes With Oral Phosphate Supplements," *Journal of Clinical Investigation*, 51 (1972, 28-34.

LANTIGUA, R., et al., "Cardiac Arrythmias Associated with a Liquid Protein Diet for the Treatment of Obesity," *New England Journal of Medicine*, 303 (1980), 735–738.

LAUER, R. M., et al., "Blood Pressure, Salt Preference, Salt Threshold and Relative Weight," *American Journal of Diseases of Childhood*, 130 (1976), 493–497.

LAWRENCE, J., et al., "Osteoarthritis." *Annals of Rheumatic Disease*, 25 (1966), 1.

LEE, C. J., et al., "Effects of Supplementation of the Diets with Calcium and Calcium-Rich Foods on Bone Density of Elderly Females with Osteoporosis." *American Journal of Clinical Nutrition*, 34 (1981), 819.

LICATA, A. A., et al., "Acute Effects of Dietary Protein on Calcium Metabolism in Patients with Osteoporosis," *Journal of Gerontology*, 36 (1) (1981), 14–19.

LINKSWEILER, H. M., et al., "Calcium Retention of Young Adult Males as Affected by Level of Protein and Calcium Intake." *Transactions of the New York Academy of Science*, 2 (36) (1974), 333–340.

LUTWAK, L., "Nutritional Aspects of Osteoporosis," *Journal of American Geriatrics Society*, 17 (2) (1969), 115–119.

_____, "Periodontal Disease," in *Nutrition and Aging*, Ed. by M. Winick. New York: John Wiley, 1976.

MACHTEY, I. and L. QUAKMIRE, "Tocopherol in Osteoarthritis: A Controlled Pilot Study," *Journal of American Geriatrics Society*, 26 (1978), 328–330.

MANN, G. V. "The Obesity Spook," *American Journal of Public Health*, 61 (1971), 1491–1498.

_____, "The Influence of Obesity in Health," *New England Journal of Medicine*, 291 (Part I) (1974), 178–185, 291 (Part II) (1974), 226–232.

_____, "Diet-Heart Hypothesis: End of an Era," New England Journal of Medicine, 297 (1977), 644–650.

_____, et al., "The Health and Nutritional Status of Eskimos," American Journal of Clinical Nutrition, 11 (1962), 31–76.

MAZESS, R. B. and R. W. MATHER, "Bone Mineral Content of North Alaskan Eskimos." *American Journal of Clinical Nutrition*, 27 (1974), 916–925.

_____, "Bone Mineral Content in Canadian Eskimos." *Human Biology*, 47 (1975), 45–63.

McGINTY, M. D., "Hiatal Hernia," *Hospital Medicine*, 7 (1971), 133–143.

McKEOWN, F., *Pathology of the Aged*, London: Butterworth's, 1965.

McMICHAEL, J., "Dietetic Factors in Coronary Disease," *European Journal of Cardiology*, 5/6 (1977), 447–452.

MERTIN, J., "Letter: Polyunsaturated Fatty Acids and Cancer," *British Medical Journal*, 4 (1973), 357.

MICHOCKI, R. J. and P. P. LAMY, "The Problem of Pressure Sores in a Nursing Home Population: Statistical Data." *Journal of American Geriatrics Society*, 24, No. 7 (1976), 323–328.

MIRANDA, P. M. and D. L. HOROWITZ, "High-Fiber Diets in the Treatment of Diabetes Mellitus," *Annals Internal Medicine*, 88 (1978), 482–486.

MITCHELL, H. S., et al., *Nutrition in Health and Disease: Handicapping Problems, Self Feeding, Chewing and Swallowing.* New York: Lippincott, 1976.

MORGAN, T., et al., "Hypertension Treated by Salt Restriction," *Lancet*, 1, (1978), 227–230.

MORRIS, J. N., et al., "Vigorous Exercise in Leisure Time and Incidence of Coronary Heart Disease," *Lancet*, 1 (1973), 333–339.

National Heart and Lung Institute. Task Force on Atherosclerosis, *A Report by the National Heart and Lung Institute Task Force, III.* Washington, D.C., National Heart and Lung Institute, 1971.

NEWBERNE, P. M., "Diet and Nutrition," *Bulletin of the New York Academy of*

Medicine, 54, No. 4 (1978), 385–396.

NEWBURGH, L. H. and J. W. CONN, "A New Interpretation of Hyperglycemia in Obese Middle Aged Persons." *Journal of the American Medical Association*, 112 (1939), 7–11.

OACE, S., "Diet and Cancer," *Journal of Nutrition Education*, 10, No. 3 (1978), 106–108.

ODLAND, L. M., et al., "Bone Density and Dietary Findings of 469 Tennesse Subjects II." *American Journal of Clinical Nutrition*, 25 (1972), 908–911.

PAFFENBURGER, R. S., et al., "Work Energy Level: Personal Characteristics and Fatal Heart Attack: A Birth Cohort Effect," *American Journal of Epidemiology*, 95 (1977), 26–37.

PAINTER, N. S. and D. P. BURKITT, "Diverticular Disease of the Colon: A Deficiency Disease of Western Civilization," *British Journal of Medicine*, 2 (1971), 707–708, 773.

PEARSE, M. L. and S. DAYTON, "Incidence of Cancer in Men on a Diet High in Polyunsaturated Fat," *Lancet* 1, 7697 (1971), 464–67.

PETO, R., "Can Dietary Beta-Carotene Materially Reduce Human Cancer Rates?" *Nature*, 290 (1981), 201–208.

PHILLIPS, R. L., "Role of Life-Styles and Dietary Habits in Risk of Cancer Among Seventh-Day Adventists," *Cancer Research*, 35 (1975), 3513–3522.

PINEL, C., "Pressure Sores," *Nursing Times*, 724 (1976), 172–174.

PIOROLA, R. C. and C. S. LIEBER, "The Energy Cost of the Metabolism of Drugs, Including Ethanol," *Pharmacology*, 7 (1972), 185–196.

PONKA, J. L., et al., "Acute Abdominal Pain in Aged Patients: An Analysis of 200 Cases," *Journal of the American Geriatrics Society*, 11 (1963), 993–1007.

POON-KING, T., et al., "The Prevalence and Natural History of Diabetes in Trinidad," *Lancet*, 1, (1968), 155–60.

PRICE, J. H. and C. PRITTS, "Overweight and Obesity in the Elderly," 1980 *Journal Gerontological Nursing*, 6:341–347.

PRIOR, I. A. M., "Diabetes in the South Pacific," in *Is the Risk of Becoming A Diabetic Affected by Sugar Consumption?* Ed. by S. S. Hildebrand. Bethesda, Maryland: International Sugar Research Foundation, 1974, p. 4–13.

RECKER, R. R. et al., "Effect of Estrogens and Calcium Carbonate on Bone Loss in Postmenopausal Women," *Annals of Internal Medicine*, 87 (1977), 649–655.

REDDY, B. S. et al., "Nutrition and Its Relationship to Cancer," *Advances in Cancer Research*, 32 (1980), 237–345.

REDDY, B. S., and E. L. WYNDER, "Large Bowel Carcinogenesis: Fecal Constituents of Populations with Diverse Incidence Rates of Colonic Cancer," *Journal of National Cancer Institute*, 50 (1973), 1437–1442.

REISER, R., "Oversimplification of Diet Coronary Heart Disease Relationships and Exaggerated Diet Recommendations," *American Journal of Clinical Nutrition*, 31 (1978), 865–875.

ROE, D., "Nutritional Concern in the Alcoholic," *Journal of American Dietetic Association*, 98 (1981), 17–21.

ROSE, G. et al., "Colon Cancer and Blood Cholesterol," *The Lancet*, 1, (1974), 7850:181–183.

SALANS, L. B., et al., "Studies on Human Adipose Tissue: Adipose Cell Life and Number in Non-obese and Obese Patients." *Journal of Clinical Investigation*, 52 (1973), 929–931.

SCHAEFER, O., "Medical Observations and Problems in the Canadian Arctic," *Canadian Medical Association Journal*, 81 (1959), 386–393.

SCHUETTE, S. A. et al., "Studies on the Mechanism of Protein Induced Hyper-Calcuria in Older Men and Women," *Journal of Nutrition*, 110 (1980), 305.

SHEKELLE, R. B.,   et al., "Dietary Vitamin A and the Risk of Cancer in the Western Electric Study," *The Lancet*, 2, (1981), 1185–1189.

SLOVIK, D. M.,   et al., "Deficient Production of 1,25-Dihydroxyvitamin D in Elderly Osteoporatic Patients," *New England Journal of Medicine*, 305 No. 7 (1981), 372–374.

SMITH, D. M.,   et al., "Age and Effects on Rare of Bone Mineral Loss," *Journal of Clinical Investigation*, 58 (1976), 716–721.

SMITH, R. W. and J. RIZEK,   "Epidemiologic Studies of Osteoporosis in Puerto Rico and Southeastern Michigan with Special Reference to Age, Race and National Origins and to Other Related or Associated Findings." *Clinical Orthopedics and Related Reserach*, 45 (1966), 31.

SPORN, M. B. and D. L. NEWTON,   "Chemoprevention of Cancer with Retinoids" *Federation Proceedings*, 38 (1979), 2528–2534.

SWEET, R.,   "Parkinson's Disease: Current Diagnosis and Treatment," in *Neurologic and Sensory Disorders in the Elderly*, Ed. by W. Fields. New York: Stratton International, 1975.

TARGOVNIK, J.,   "Senile Osteoporosis," *Arizona Medicine*, 34, No. 8 (1977), 543–544.

TROWELL, H. C.,   "Dietary-Fiber Hypothesis of the Etiology of Diabetes Mellitus," *Diabetes*, 24 (1975), 762–765.

_____, "Definition of Dietary Fiber and Hypotheses that It's a Protective Factor in Certain Diseases," *American Journal of Clinical Nutrition*, 29 (1976), 417–427.

_____, "Diabetes Mellitus and Dietary Fiber of Starchy Foods," *American Journal of Clinical Nutrition*, 31 (1978), 553–557.

USDHEW, *Third Special Report to the U.S. Congress on Alcohol and Health*, Washington: U.S. Department of Health, Education and Welfare, 1978.

USPHS, *Diabetes Data*. Bethesda, Maryland: U.S. Department of Health, Education and Welfare, 1978.

VISICK, W. J.,   *Evidence Supporting the Hypothesis that Ammonia Increases Cancer*. Ithaca: Cornell University, (unpublished ms.), 1975.

WALKER, A. R. P.,   "Sugar Intake and Coronary Heart Disease." *Atherosclerosis*, 14 (1971), 137.

_____, "Dietary Fiber and Pattern of Disease," *Annals of Internal Medicine*, 80 (1974), 663–664.

_____ and D.P. BURKITT,   "Colonic Cancer—Hypothesis of Causation, Dietary Prophylaxis and Future Research," *American Journal of Digestive Diseases*, 21:1976, 910–917.

WEG, R.,   *Nutrition and the Later Years*. Los Angeles: University of Southern California Press, 1978.

WHEDON, G. D.,   "Recent Advances in Management of Osteoporosis," in *Phosphate and Minerals in Health and Disease*, Ed. by S. G. Massry, et al., New York: Plenum, 1980.

WINICK, M,   *Nutrition in Health and Disease*. New York: John Wiley, 1981.

WYNDER, E. L. and G. B. GORI,   "Contribution of the Environment to Cancer Incidence. *Journal of National Cancer Institute*, 58 (1977), 825–833.

YOUNG, V. R. and P. M. NEWBERNE,   "Vitamins and Cancer Prevention: Issues and Dilemmas," *Cancer*, 47 (1981), 1226–1240.

YUDKIN, J. M.,   "Dietary Fat and Dietary Sugar in Relation to Ischaemic Heart Disease and Diabetes," *Lancet*, 2, (1969), 4–5.

_____, *Pure White and Deadly*. London Davis-Poynter, 1972.

CHAPTER SEVEN
NUTRITION, THE
AGED, AND SOCIETY

If one were seriously interested in writing a history of government programs for the aged in America, a good starting point would probably be late sixteenth century England where *systematic* policies for dealing with dependent individuals gradually began to be implemented. In 1598, during the reign of Elizabeth I, an act of relief for the poor was passed. These famous Poor Laws, precipitated by economic and political changes in sixteenth century England, attempted to distinguish among the various categories of the needy. They provided for "the necessary relief of the lame, impotent, old, blind, and such other being poor and not able to work." One consequence of the Poor Laws was the development of so-called poorhouses to house and feed the incapacitated and/or aged poor without families, and to assume responsibility for them. The principles embodied in the laws were retained for almost 250 years and for the duration acted to direct policies in America as well as in England regarding all dependent people including those who were aged.

The poorhouse environment was generally harsh and punitive. It quite accurately reflected the hostility and fear toward those old and poor who were disaffiliated from kith and kin. Persons accused of witchcraft during the sixteenth and seventeenth centuries in England were characteristically middle-aged or old, very likely to be widowed, and poor (MacFarlane, 1970). Such people, the long-lived especially, were deemed to have mysterious power.

Crocker (1974) suggests it is no coincidence that in this period of accusations of witchcraft, specialty institutions for housing the old and poor were developed.

American colonists followed the English model closely and thus American poor laws were quite consistent with those of England. If American poor laws differed, it was because an ethic of individualism influenced them. (Mencher, 1967). By the middle of the eighteenth century, most urban areas had established all-purpose institutions to handle the poor, old, and disaffiliated. In the early part of the nineteenth century, poorhouses were quite common in almost all settled areas of the United States with the notable exception of the deep south.

It is important to remember the prevailing social values that were fundamental to the implementation of Poor Laws and to the development of all-purpose poorhouses. Poverty, or public dependency of any kind, was tantamount to moral degeneracy and thus required a similar response on the part of society. Poverty resulting from mental or physical illness was not differentiated from poverty resulting from widowhood or any other vagary of old age. According to one historian who studied relief of the poor in Massachusetts:

> Poverty was not differentiated from chronic pauperism and pauperism was akin to crime. The sturdy beggar, the idiot, the drunkard, and the widow who was only poor were herded together under the same roof, the chief source of anxiety being the net cost of the establishment (Kelso, 1922:101, quoted in Crocker, 1974).

Children were the first to be removed from the poorhouse setting to separate institutions. This exception appears to have begun in the late eighteenth century and was practiced almost universally by the latter part of the nineteenth century. Children were not held guilty of immorality themselves and removal from the poorhouse was thought to prevent life-long "contamination." As Crocker (1974) points out, the principle of differentiating those of the dependent who could not be held responsible for their conditions, which was first inaugurated for children, was applied successively to the insane, the feeble-minded, the deaf, dumb, blind, and epileptics. This separation of categories of individuals from the poorhouse occurs through the nineteenth century and into the twentieth. By default, the elderly were relegated to and remained in the poorhouse. Approximately 70 percent of the elderly institutionalized in the U.S. were in poorhouses in 1904; the figure for 1910 decreased to 57 percent (Manard, Kart and van Gils, 1975).

However, by the latter part of the nineteenth century and early into the twentieth, a new attitude toward caring for the aged seemed to be emerging. Perhaps stimulated by the changing demographics of modern societies, an increased life expectancy, a growing older population, and/or economic depression, people began to see old age as a social problem (Maddox and Wiley,

1976). Recognizing the prevalence of incapacity, isolation, and poverty among aged citizens, western society's concern turned toward social action on behalf of the aged (Burgess, 1960). This concern and the accompanying perceived need for collective social action was reflected in governmental legislation.

In 1889, Germany created a system of social insurance which included a pension scheme. For the first time, the aged were given a measure of economic security as a right rather than as charity. In Denmark, state support for needy old people was introduced in 1891. Pension rights were introduced in Great Britain in 1908 for people over the age of seventy who had been in regular employment but had little or no income after leaving their job.

During the early part of this century and into the 1920s, continuing attempts were made in the United States to define pensions as a right of aged Americans. These attempts met with limited success. Several states enacted old-age pension legislation, and reform groups such as the American Association of Old Age Security began to appear. The Great Depression, with its devastating economic impact on the lives of many Americans, helped create conditions that ultimately allowed the enactment of federal legislation promoting the pension rights of the aged and ensuring unemployment insurance.

Unemployment during the depression was in excess of 25 percent among the elderly. Bank failures and the declining value of estates exhausted financial resources of millions including even those among the more prosperous middle and upper-middle classes. In 1932, the American Federation of Labor reversed its previous position and endorsed unemployment insurance and old-age assistance at the state and federal levels.

Utopian schemes were prevalent during this period, exemplified by Upton Sinclair's EPIC ("end poverty in California") plan and the "ham and eggs" movement also based in California (Fischer, 1977). Perhaps the most popular of these utopian schemes was that put forth by Dr. Francis Townsend of Long Beach, California. The essence of the Townsend plan was that all Americans over sixty would receive a monthly sum of $200 on the condition that they spent this pension money within thirty days. A 2 percent tax on all business transactions was to pay for the plan (Achenbaum, 1978). By 1936, Townsend claimed a national following of over five million and at least sixty congressmen sympathetic to this measure (Putnam, 1970).

Clearly, the idea of an old-age pension in America had achieved legitimacy. The institutional structure needed to implement this idea was the Social Security Act of 1935. With its passage, the United States became one of the last industrial nations to establish a federal old-age pension program. Since then, though, chronological age has increasingly been used as the basis upon which to allocate the benefits of government programs. As Kutza (1981) points out, in America today there is a federal system of old-age pensions (Social Security), a guaranteed annual income program for older persons (Supplemental Security Income), a national health insurance plan for the elderly (Medicare), senior citizen housing, and a comprehensive social services planning and coordinating system for the aged (Older Americans Act). Estes (1979) has identified at least eighty programs in the *1978 Catalog of Federal Domestic Assistance* that were of benefit to the aged directly or indirectly. In contradiction to rhetoric sometimes heard about government ignoring the plight of the elderly, it would seem that the aged have become a favored social welfare constituency in the U.S.

Robert Hudson (1978) distinguishes between "breakthrough" and "constituency-building" policy enactments which may bring favored status upon a special interest group. Breakthrough policies consist of those pieces of legislation that involve the federal government in providing or guaranteeing some fundamental benefit. Constituency-building policies are those that recognize that different groups have common interest and allow "space" for these interest groups in the making of public policy. The aged have been principal beneficiaries and a functional constituency in the federal government's involvement in breakthrough legislation to ensure health care financing for high risk populations (for example, Medicare and Medicaid) and to guarantee minimum income for the impoverished (for example, Supplemental Security Income) (Hudson, 1978).

Another perspective involves making the distinction between programs *for* the elderly and those that *affect* the elderly. So-called age-entitlement programs, including Social Security and Medicare, for example, base eligibility for benefits directly upon age and can be described as being *for* the elderly. Food stamps and public housing, which are programs that determine eligibility on the basis of financial need and which are sometimes referred to as need-entitlement programs, are examples of programs that *affect* the elderly. A third category of programs beneficial to many of the elderly includes government initiatives that affect nearly all people regardless of age or need. Taxation practices, regulatory activities, and monetary policies are examples of government initiatives which may affect the elderly even more profoundly than programs aimed directly at them (Katza, 1981).

In the following pages, five federal programs benefiting the elderly indirectly or directly will be briefly described. Two of these, the Food Stamp program and Title III (formerly Title VII) of the Older Americans Act have specific missions to maintain or improve nutritional status. Three other programs, colloquially referred to as Social Security (including SSI), Medicare (Title XVIII of the Social Security Act), and public housing contribute directly to maintaining or increasing the income, health, and housing status of elderly Americans and thus have significant impact on nutritional status. These programs represent a mix of age- and need-entitlement and, with the exception of Social Security, which provides a direct cash benefit, provide indirect benefits (benefits-in-kind).

PROGRAMS BENEFITING
THE ELDERLY

The Food Stamp Program

During the 1930s, agricultural economists became interested in commodity distribution plans (some that involved the use of food coupons) in order to expand market demand for agricultural products. It was generally believed that such programs could help dispose of surplus agricultural commodities, provide income subsidies for farm families, and improve the nutritional status of low-income families. The war effort slowed development of these plans, but in 1949 Congress passed an Agricultural Act that directed the Secretary of Agriculture to distribute commodities acquired through federal price supports to low-income families. Trattner (1979) suggests that this commodity scheme was designed primarily to promote the interests of farmers rather than those of poor consumers since it depended entirely on the availability of surplus foods, and not on the nutritional needs of poor Americans.

In response to deficiencies in the commodities distribution program, the Food Stamp Program was initiated in 1961 as a pilot project in eight areas by executive order of President Kennedy. By 1964, food stamp projects were operating in 22 states. The pilot program was institutionalized with the Food Stamp Act of 1964. This legislation represented a compromise between proponents of a food program for the poor and the interests of agricultural producers. Congress intended the act "to promote the general welfare, that the nation's abundance of food should be utilized cooperatively by the States, the Federal Government, and local government units to the maximum extent practicable to safeguard the health and raise the levels of nutrition among low-income households (Schmandt, Shorey and Kinch, 1980)."

As it was initially conceived, the program allowed households with income below the poverty line to purchase food stamps at a discount. In theory, the face value of purchased stamps would be sufficient to allow a household to purchase enough items for an adequate, nutritional diet. Food would be obtained through normal marketing outlets (giant supermarkets or "ma and pa" convenience stores) and it was expected that retail food stores would redeem the stamps at face value. Nonfood items such as cigarettes, alcoholic beverages, or pet food could not be purchased with the stamps.

Presently, the number of stamps each eligible household receives is determined by the dollar amount required to purchase a "Thrifty Food Plan" as determined by the Department of Agriculture for various family sizes. The Thrifty Plan exceeds the nutritional goal of recommended daily allowances by five percent for food energy, protein, calcium, iron, vitamin A value, thiamine, riboflavin, niacin, and ascorbic acid. Fat provides no more than 40 percent of the food energy (USDHEW, 1976).

It is assumed that a family should be able to allocate 30 percent of its income toward the purchase of food. For example, a family of four with a monthly net income of $300 can be expected to contribute $90 toward food purchases. If, according to the USDA, a Thrifty Food Plan for a family of four can be purchased for $170, the family is eligible for an allotment of stamps worth $80. Prior to amendments to the Food Stamp Act in 1977, recipients bought the food stamps at a price below cash value. Families in the lowest economic groups paid nothing, but the price of the stamps rose with income. Thus the family in the above example would purchase $170 in food stamps for $90. The effect of the 1977 change was to allow participation by households who could not afford the monthly purchase requirement. Thus, beginning in 1978, the family in our example simply received an $80 allotment of food stamps. The elimination of the purchase requirement is generally believed to have increased participation in the program. Most households eligible for food stamps probably spend additional cash to purchase an adequate diet. In addition, it must be noted that the food stamp program cannot ensure that participating families consume nutritionally adequate diets, only that they possess sufficient funds to purchase one.

When the program was begun in 1964, only 360,000 people were participating at a federal cost of $28.6 million (Sexauer, 1977). While the original Food Stamp Act of 1964 provided for federal and state participation with administrative costs shared on a 50/50 matching basis, not all states participated. Texas, for example, did not enter the program until 1970. It is estimated that in fiscal year 1981, food stamps worth $9.7 billion were distributed to over 20 million persons (Special Committee on Aging, 1980). Estimates vary as to the number of elderly participants in the program. A Department of Agriculture survey in 1976 found one or more elderly persons in 17 percent of food stamp households surveyed, and the total number of elderly persons receiving food stamps was estimated at just below one million (USDA, 1977). About half of these elderly recipients were living alone and the majority of single-person households were occupied by women.

According to one observer (Sexauer, 1977), the food stamp program has helped to significantly reduce chronic hunger in America. Others have noted the growing importance of the program's "income maintenance" function. Increasingly, the program has reached the poor and working poor who were not eligible for other forms of income support (MacDonald, 1977). A 1977 Congressional Budget Office report calls Food Stamps the "only national program providing assistance to all needy families."

Title III of the Older Americans Act

While commodity distribution and food stamps were available to some of the elderly in the mid-1960s, it was generally recognized that they did not meet the specific nutritional needs of "high risk" groups of elderly—the sick, the poor, minorities, and the socially isolated. In response to the needs of these elderly people, the Administration on Aging, established under the U.S. Department of Health, Education, and Welfare (now Health and Human Services) by the Older Americans Act (OAA) of 1965, conducted research and demonstration projects to improve the nutritional status of elderly Americans. Beginning in 1968, the Congress provided annual funds (for three years) for those projects.

One objective of the projects was to develop methods for providing nutritionally adequate and appetizing meals for the elderly in congregate settings. They also sought to combat problems that seemed to increase nutritional vulnerability such as poor nutrition education, ill health, social isolation, and lack of transportation. By 1971, 32 demonstration projects had met with considerable success in their operations across the U.S.

While no formal quantitative evaluation of the demonstration projects was ever completed, their popularity with the public seemed to provide an impetus for the passage of legislation to expand service delivery to the elderly in general, with the congregate meals program receiving particular attention. In 1973, Congress passed the Comprehensive Services Amendments to the Older Americans Act. Among these amendments was Title VII, which provided formula grants to the states to pay a substantial part of the cost of establishing and operating low-cost meal programs for people 60 years of age and older. The programs were to be located in community settings such as schools, senior citizen centers, and churches easily accessible to the elderly. One hot meal a day was provided at least five days during the week, along with other services intended to introduce participants to social resources in the community. Participants were expected to pay a nominal fee for each meal, and meals could be delivered to older persons who were homebound (Meenaghan and Washington, 1980). The formal goals of the program are listed in Table 7.1.

By some standards the Title VII program was an enormous success. Through the first quarter of 1978 over $620 million had been expended on the delivery of Title VII services. In fact, the largest appropriation for any program in the Older Americans Act was for nutrition services (Estes, 1979). According to the Special Committee on Aging of the U.S. Senate (1979), there were 9,732 nutrition sites operating during 1978 under the administration of 1,074 nutrition projects. Approximately 470,000 meals were served each day—83 percent in congregate, community settings and 17 percent to the

TABLE 7.1.   Goals of national nutrition programs for the elderly.

1. Improve the health of the elderly with the provision of regularly available low-cost nutritious meals served largely in congregate settings and when feasible, to the homebound.
2. Increase the incentive of elderly persons to maintain social well-being by providing opportunities for social interaction and the satisfying use of leisure time.
3. Improve the capability of the elderly to prepare meals at home by providing auxiliary services including nutrition and homemaker education, shopping assistance, and transportation to markets.
4. Increase the incentive of the elderly to maintain good health and independent living by providing counseling and information and referral to other social and rehabilitation services.
5. Assure that those of the elderly most in need, primarily the low-income, minorities, and the isolated, can and do participate in nutrition services by providing an extensive and personalized outreach program and transportation service.
6. Stimulate minority elderly interest in nutrition services by assuring them that operation of the projects reflects cultural pluralism in both the meal and supportive service components.
7. Assure that program participants have access to a comprehensive and coordinated system of services by encouraging administration coordination between nutrition projects and area agencies on aging.

Source: U.S. Department of Health, Education, and Welfare, Committee on Research and Development, Gerontological Society. *Evaluative Research on Social Programs for the Elderly*. Washington, D.C.: Government Printing Office, 1973, p. 142.

homebound—and at many sites the number of people on waiting lists were twice that of the number of meals being served daily. The committee reports more than 1.5 million persons (two-thirds of these were low-income) were served meals at the nutrition sites, though this data is difficult to evaluate. Kutza (1981) reports that while Illinois officials estimated that 1.4 million elderly received major services through the Older Americans Act in the state, no one knew how much double counting this estimate reflected. That is, no one could say how many persons were getting more than one service and/or how many services were being given to the same person more than once.

Despite the growth and apparent success of Title VII programs, some criticism has been directed at them. Posner (1979) suggests that, virtually from its birth, Title VII shifted away from any provision of related health or supportive services to a singular concentration on the delivery of meals. According to her, only about 13 percent of total program costs ever went for social services. Lakoff (1976) argues that this deviation from the long-term goals of the program was related to shorter-term political motives. After all, the goals of "stimulating interest" and "increasing incentives" are not as tangible as delivering meals, which is an easily quantifiable service that has clear visibility. Other concerns included the sometimes bitter power struggles between area agencies on aging and the formerly independent nutrition projects, the effect of the program's universal eligibility requirements, and the level of assistance the program provided in relation to actual need (Estes, 1979). By 1977 one author could write that the opportunity to develop the program's position as the vanguard of national health efforts for the aged had not been accomplished (Watkin, 1977).

In response to these concerns and others (for example, duplication of services, lack of coordination), Congress again, in 1978, amended the Older Americans Act. Its revised purpose was to foster "the development of comprehensive and coordinated service systems to serve older individuals," and it had an expanded mission "to provide a continuum of care for the vulnerable elderly." Virtually all social and nutrition service (including Title VII) were consolidated under a *new* Title III. Specifically identified services include health, continuing education, welfare, information and referral, recreation, homemaker, counseling, transportation, housing, alternatives to institutionalization, legal, tax and financial, physical activity, and preretirement. Authorizations for senior centers and ombudsman services were also included under the new title.

Title III authorizes the continuation of congregate nutrition programs that provide at least "one hot or other appropriate meal" 5 days or more each week to persons 60 years of age and older. Each meal is expected to account for at least one-third of the daily recommended dietary allowances. The law also allows each nutrition project to provide nutrition education and other appropriate nutritional services for its participants. For the first time, the home-delivered meals program for the elderly received a separate authorization. It requires each project to provide at least five meals per week which are "hot, cold, frozen, dried, canned, or supplemental foods (with a satisfactory storage life)," and each meal should again account for at least one-third of the daily recommended dietary allowances.

The total 1981 fiscal year budget (congregate and home delivered meals) was expected to maintain a level of daily meals served of 410,000, which is below the figure reported earlier for 1978. Approximately 57,000 of these meals were to be delivered to the homebound elderly (Special Committee on Aging, 1980). Actual requests of $340 million for fiscal 1981 were considerably below the ceiling level of $520 million authorized in the 1978 amendments. At the time of this writing, the status of Title III (and other programs subsumed under the Older Americans Act) in the first Reagan (1982) budget is still unclear.

Social Security

The Social Security Act of 1935 established a federal old-age pension program (OAI) and a federal-state system of unemployment insurance. The original legislation was strengthened and expanded in 1939 when survivors' and dependents' benefits were added (OASI). Disability insurance (OASDI) was added in 1956 and Medicare (OASDHI) became operative in 1965. More changes were made in 1972, including the automatic cost-of-living adjustment of benefits and the establishment of Supplemental Security Income (SSI) as a replacement for aid to the indigent, blind, and disabled (see below).

In 1948 only 13 percent of all persons sixty-five years and over were receiving social security payments. Since then, additional groups of workers have been brought into the system. In 1950, 64.5 percent of all paid employment positions were covered under social security. This number had increased to 90 percent by 1972 (Gold, Kutza, and Marmor, 1977). In 1974, the railroad retirement program was integrated into the system. Currently, in excess of nine out of ten American workers are covered, and over 90 percent of the elderly receive some income support through the social security system.

The old age, survivors, and disability program (OASDI) is the single largest program in the federal budget, and in 1981 it was expected to pay out $136.9 billion to almost 36 million beneficiaries—$91.1 billion of this amount was earmarked for the aged. The projected beneficiaries include 19.8 million retired workers, 2.9 million disabled, and 13.2 million dependents and survivors (Special Committee on Aging, 1980).

Social security eligibility is related to work rather than need. In 1979 a person was credited with a quarter of coverage for each $260 earned during the year, with a maximum of four quarters of coverage in a given year. Under current stipulation of the law, a person who will reach age sixty-two in 1983 needs thirty-two quarters to achieve minimum eligibility for retirement benefits. A person who reaches age sixty-two in 1991 or later would need forty quarters of coverage to be eligible.

Benefits are financed by payroll taxes paid equally by employees and employers on earned income up to a certain level (self-employed persons are taxed individually on their earnings). In 1982 this tax is 13.40 percent (6.70 percent withheld from employees) on the first $31,800. This is scheduled to increase to 13.40 percent on the first $33,900 in 1983. Thus the maximum tax paid by an employee in 1982 is $2,130.60. In 1983 it will increase to $2,271.30.

Retirement benefits are paid to persons who have worked for a minimum period of time on one or more "covered" jobs and who can be considered "substantially" retired. The Social Security Administration employs a "retirement test" to determine whether or not a person otherwise eligible for retirement benefits can be considered retired. Essentially, the retirement test acts to reduce benefits paid persons under age seventy-two who earn more than a certain amount. For example, a sixty-eight year old man could earn up to $6,000 in 1982 without any reduction in social security benefits. Benefits are reduced one dollar for every two dollars earned above the exempt amount.

For the first half of 1979, the minimum retirement benefit for a worker at age sixty-five was $1,416.60 a year. This could be raised to $2,276.00 for one who has achieved thirty years or more of covered employment. Maximum benefits are limited by a ceiling placed on earnings on which the worker had made contributions. In January of 1979, the maximum retirement benefit payable to a worker who was sixty-five was $6,040.80 a year. The average monthly benefit level in July 1980 was $330 for a retired worker, $538 for a retired couple, and $305 for an aged widow or widower. This low average benefit level reflects the fact that over one-half of current social security recipients *do not* receive full benefits. This is in part due to the popularity of the early retirement option.

Early retirement benefits may be paid to people who retire between ages sixty-two and sixty-four. These benefits are reduced (approximately 20 percent) to take into account the longer period over which they will be paid. Delayed benefit credits are also available. Up until 1979, benefits were increased one percent for each year after 1970 in which the worker between sixty-five and seventy-two did not receive any benefits. For those reaching sixty-two in 1979 (and beyond) an additional three percent will be added to benefits for each year between sixty-five and seventy-two that benefits are not received.

Munnell (1977) has evaluated the "replacement rate" structure of social security benefits and finds it to be quite progressive. "Replacement rate" refers to the proportion of preretirement income provided by social security. In general, it appears that as the earnings record of a worker rises, the social security replacement rate falls. However, Fox (1979) reports that the median social security replacement rates for 1973–74 retirees varied between 32 and 49 percent.

Social security has had enormous impact in reducing the extent of poverty among the aged. In 1966, 60 percent of social security benefits went to people who would have been below the poverty line without such benefits. This has led at least one economist to characterize social security as the most successful social program in the history of the country (Hollister, 1974).

The influence of social security as a retirement pension system is difficult to overestimate (Calhoun, 1978). As one historian of aging in America has pointed out, the Social Security Act of 1935: (1) established the principle of a guaranteed "floor" income as a right bought by contributions over the course of a working life; (2) gave added impetus to demands for the extension of private pension coverage; (3) provided a standard age by which retirement could be defined; and (4) signaled a new era in financial arrangements for life after retirement (Calhoun, 1978).

Current questions about the social security system concern its financial status. During its early years of existence, more revenue was taken in from contributions than was paid out in benefits, and a trust fund was developed. By 1976, this situation had changed. Boskin (1977) estimates that social security was paying out $4.3 billion more in 1976 than was being taken in. At that rate, the trust fund would probably have run out during the mid-1980s. Payroll taxes have been increased (as well as the maximum taxable income level) to offset this situation. But this may not be a long-term solution, especially during extended periods of inflation, economic slowdown, and/or high unemployment. Many believe these taxes to be too high already and the demographic factors that have contributed to the trust fund's deficit are not likely to disappear. These factors include the aging of the population, the shift to early retirement, and the increasing length of the average period of retirement.

Numerous proposals have been put forth for dealing with the long-term financial problems of social security. Among them are the reduction of early retirement benefits, raising the retirement age to 68, elimination of "minimum" social security benefits, and a reforming of the automatic inflation adjustment introduced in 1972. Each proposal raises complex issues of equity. Devising a solution to the current problems will require an overall examination of the goals and design of the program.

Supplemental Security Income. Included in the Social Security Act of 1935 was a mandate for the establishment of a separate program of old-age assistance under which benefits (coming mostly from federal funds) would be distributed to the needy among the aged and administered by the states. Similar programs for the blind and disabled were established in the 1935 Act and subsequent amendments. Under the Social Security Amendments of 1972, a new federal program of Supplemental Security Income (SSI) for the aged, blind, and disabled replaced the former state-operated welfare programs. This new program became effective January 1, 1974.

The SSI program was envisioned as a basic national income maintenance system for the aged, blind, and disabled (U.S. Senate Committee on Finance, 1977). The program was expected to supplement the social security program primarily by providing income support to those not covered by social security. Applicants to this program must prove need by meeting an "assets test."

Federal benefit payments for SSI during fiscal year 1981 are expected to reach $6.1 billion for approximately 4.2 million needy aged, blind, and disabled persons. Over 1.5 million of these individuals are aged. The maximum federal payment level under SSI was estimated to reach $259 per month for eligible individuals and $388 per month for eligible couples after July 1, 1981 (Special Committee on Aging, 1980). Many states provide an additional supplement to the federal benefit. Any unearned income over $20 a month reduces the benefit dollar for dollar, and monthly wages over $85 reduce it by 50 cents for each dollar of earned income.

Medicare

In 1965, the Social Security Act of 1935 was amended to provide health insurance for the elderly. This amendment, which became effective July 1, 1966, is known as Title XVIII or Medicare. It marked the inauguration in America of a national system of financing individual health services. In 1972, Title XVIII extended benefits to two other groups that have severe difficulty in paying for medical care—the disabled and persons suffering from chronic kidney disease.

The passage of Medicare was the culmination of an almost century-long effort by proponents of national health insurance. For example, in the first decades of this century the American Association for Labor Legislation, an organization of academics, lawyers, and other professionals, attempted to pass a "model" medical care insurance bill through several state legislatures. They had no success. The American Medical Association opposed the bills as did the American Federation of Labor. The AMA feared "socialized medicine" while the AFL feared "government control of the workers."

While advocates of compulsory health insurance annually proposed bills in Congress from 1939 on, it was not until Truman's "Fair Deal" that the possibilities of passing such a bill become strong. In 1949 President Truman requested congressional action on medical care insurance. In order to placate the AMA, the "Blues" and commercial insurance carriers, it was specified that doctors and hospitals would not have to join the program. However, there was still opposition and despite Truman's characterization of the AMA as "the public's worst enemy in the efforts to redistribute medical care more equitably," efforts at passing a national health insurance bill were defeated (Marmor, 1973).

Clearly, another strategy was necessary. The one that developed involved turning away from the health problems of the general population to those of the aged. There was great appeal in focusing on the aged. As a group, they were needy yet deserving, and most had made a contribution to America. Yet through no fault of their own, many suffered reduced earning capacity and higher medical expenses. Proponents of this new strategy waged a public war of sympathy for the aged and a private war of pressure politics from 1952 to 1965. Not until then was the political climate ripe for amending the original Social Security Act to provide health insurance for America's aged.

Medicare consists of two basic components. Part A is a compulsory hospital insurance plan that covers a bed patient in a hospital and, under certain conditions, in a skilled nursing facility or at home after having left the hospital. It is financed by employer-employee payroll tax contributions and a tax on the self-employed. Part A coverage is near-universal with about 99 percent of all aged persons enrolled.

Part B represents a voluntary program of supplemental medical insurance that helps pay doctor bills, outpatient hospital benefits, home health services, and certain other medical services and supplies. Financing is achieved through monthly premiums paid by enrollees (about 96 percent of the aged) and matching funds by the federal government. In 1980 the monthly premium for participation in Part B was $9.60. In addition, the subscriber pays the first $60 in charges incurred in a year and 20 percent of the remainder. Although Part B pays for a broad array of services, it *does not* cover such things as routine physical examinations, foot care, eye or hearing examinations, eyeglasses or hearing aids, prescription drugs, false teeth, and full-time nursing care.

Hospital insurance (Part A) benefits are measured by periods of time known as benefit periods. Benefit periods begin when a patient enters the hospital and end when he or she has not been a hospital bed patient for sixty consecutive days. This concept is an important one, since it determines how much care a Medicare beneficiary is entitled to at any particular point in time. Medicare will help to pay for up to ninety days of in-hospital patient care, for up to 100 days of extended care in a skilled nursing facility, and for up to 100 home health visits in each benefit period. There is no limit to the number of benefit periods to which an individual is entitled. If an individual runs out of covered days within a benefit period he or she may draw upon a lifetime reserve of sixty additional hospital days. Use of these days within the lifetime reserve, however, permanently reduces the total number of reserve days left. For example, if a patient has been in the hospital for ninety days and needs ten more days of hospital care, he or she may draw ten days from the reserve of sixty, leaving him or her with a reserve of fifty days.

Part A Medicare benefits will pay for such services as a semiprivate room, including meals and special diets, regular nursing services, laboratory tests, drugs, medical supplies, and appliances furnished by the hospital. It will not pay for convenience items, a private room, private duty nurses, or doctors' services paid for through Part B.

A Medicare patient is financially responsible for various components of his or her hospital insurance plan. For example, as a bed patient in a participating hospital, an individual is responsible for the first $204 (1981 figure) of costs in each benefit period. After this, Part A pays for covered services for the first sixty days of hospital care. From the sixty-first through the ninetieth day in a benefit period, hospital insurance pays for all covered services except for $41 a day (1981 figure). If more than ninety days of inpatient care is required, an additional, higher copayment is required. All covered extended-care services are paid for for the first twenty days. After this period, the recipient must make a coinsurance payment of $25.50 a day for up to eighty additional days in a benefit period.

Estimated Part A payments for the aged in fiscal year 1981 are $22.6 billion. Total outlays for Part B for the elderly are estimated to be about $9.5 billion in 1981 (Special Committee on Aging, 1980). These figures represent a radically different picture from the past. In fiscal 1966, the year Medicare was implemented, total health care expenditures in the U.S. amounted to $42 billion or $212 per person. Total Medicare payments for the aged in 1981 (estimated at $32.1 billion) come to almost $1300 per aged person. However, Medicare alone still pays for between 40 and 45 percent of all medical care for the elderly. While this percentage varies by the type of health care purchased (for example, Medicare pays for over 70 percent of hospital care) and other public funds contribute to paying the health care bill of the elderly, out-of-pocket expenditures are still very high. Dental services, drugs, and eyeglasses are almost always paid for directly by older people. In addition, the elderly still pay out-of-pocket for 46.7 percent of nursing home costs and 40.9 percent of the cost of physician services (Kart, 1981).

Medicaid, or Title XIX of the Social Security Act, was also passed in 1965 and became effective July 1, 1966. According to Stevens and Stevens (1974), some observers at the time saw Medicaid as the "sleeper" of the 1965 legislation. Medicaid was intended as a catch-all program to handle medical expenses not covered by Medicare as well as to provide medical assistance to needy groups other than the aged. For example, Medicaid provides long-term, unlimited nursing home care without requiring previous hospitalization. Not surprisingly, Medicaid has become the principal public mechanism for funding nursing home care. Combined federal and state Medicaid payments to nursing homes are estimated at $9.4 billion in fiscal year 1981.

The Medicaid program is jointly funded by federal and state governments with the federal government contributing in excess of 50 percent in "poorer" states. Eligibility varies from one state to another, although one requirement seems to be almost universal. Wherever an individual qualifies for Medicaid, "pauperization" has preceded qualification. Persons, including the elderly, may find themselves eligible for Medicaid only after they have drained their resources and qualified as a member of "the poor."

Public Housing

Major federal involvement in housing began with the Housing Act of 1937, which was designated to meet the needs of low-income families. In 1956, this act was amended to provide public housing specifically for the elderly. Since that time, a considerable amount of construction has taken place. According to Carp (1976), under various programs of the Department of Housing and Urban Development (HUD), approximately 750,000 older people have been rehoused. About 600,000 of these live in special housing for the elderly. Though these numbers seem impressive, the need for additional housing is great. The 1971 White House Conference on Aging called for an annual production of 120,000 units of new housing for the elderly. The recently concluded 1981 White House Conference on Aging recommended providing a minimum of 200,000 units of housing each year for the elderly through the cooperative efforts of government and the private sector. One problem, as Lawton (1980) points out, is that most federal housing programs lead a precarious existence. They may be initiated and terminated within the term of one or two presidential administrations.

Most public housing construction involves low-cost, high-rise apartment buildings. To be eligible for public housing designed specifically for the elderly a person must be sixty-two years or over, or handicapped (without age restrictions). Restrictions on income and assets are usually set at the local level. Almost uniformly, tenants pay rent on a sliding scale to a maximum of

25 percent of total income. Preliminary proposals from the Reagan administration in this area suggest the possibility that this may increase to 30 or 35
percent of total income. Two continuing federal housing programs for the
elderly are Section 202 and Section 8.

Section 202.   Originally enacted as part of the Housing Act of 1959,
this program was designed to provide "independent living" for elderly and
handicapped persons. Suspended in 1968, the program was revived in 1974.
Section 202 authorizes direct loans to nonprofit organizations so that they can
develop and operate multifamily housing projects. These projects are expected
to be small-scale and aimed primarily at moderate-income elderly persons.
According to HUD (1979), the program has produced approximately 45,000
housing units in 335 projects located throughout the nation. The fiscal 1981
budget projects $830 million in loan authority to support an estimated 18,800
units of Section 202 housing. The congregate housing services program, a
demonstration program in Section 202, and public housing facilities which
supports meals, housekeeping assistance, and personal care, received no
budget request for 1981. The congress had appropriated $10 million for both
fiscal years 1979 and 1980 for such demonstrations.

Most Section 202 housing is located within cities in predominantly residential neighborhoods where there is little or no other public or subsidized
housing. The residents of these neighborhoods tend to be white, lower-to-
middle income, and nonelderly (USHUD, 1979). Aside from age, many of the
status characteristics of neighborhood residents are quite similar to those of
Section 202 tenants. The program appears to be serving primarily white,
elderly females who have middle socioeconomic status backgrounds and
current income that, while low in absolute terms, is in the moderate to middle
range of elderly incomes. Males, blacks, other minorities, the handicapped,
and persons with very low incomes appear poorly served by the program
(USHUD, 1979).

Section 8.   This program, which replaces the Section 236 mortgage
insurance program, is currently the principal federal means of providing
housing assistance to the elderly. Under this section, HUD contracts with
private developers for the leasing of units to low-income families who would
otherwise meet the eligibility requirements for public housing. HUD provides
rent supplements to these families, who pay no more than 25 percent of their
income for rent, and pays the owners the difference between fair market rent
and the amount the tenant must pay. One innovation of this program is the
flexibility given to communities for the developing of strategies to deal with
low-cost housing needs. A budget authority of $24 billion was requested by
HUD for the Section 8 rent subsidy program in fiscal 1981. HUD estimates
that approximately 258,000 reservations for housing assistance payments will
be made during 1981—120,000 for existing housing and 138,000 for new construction (Special Committee on Aging, 1980). Recent history suggests that

about 25 percent of these reservations will go either to individuals aged sixty-two or over or to elderly families.

ARE THE AGED A FAVORED CONSTITUENCY IN THE U.S.?

There is currently some considerable debate about the economic costs of programs for the elderly, especially the age-entitlement programs. Some commentators see the costs of programs for the elderly as the dominant factor shaping federal spending and taxing decisions, and one analyst has already characterized the cost of an aging America as having the potential to "bust the U.S. budget (Samuelson, 1978)."

According to Robert Samuelson (1978), spending for the elderly amounted to one-fifth of the federal budget in 1969. By 1979 this figure had increased to almost one-third of federal expenditures. Almost 80 percent of federal spending for the elderly in 1979 was funneled through social security and Medicare. Samuelson believes that there will be continued pressure on the federal budget in coming years. As the size of the elderly population increases, the government must raise taxes and reduce funding for other programs or run increasingly large deficits. In the Reagan years, a political scenario that includes sharply higher taxes seems unlikely. However, higher deficits seem unavoidable without tax increases, even in the face of significant reductions in federally sponsored social programs. Economic recession, the fight against inflation, higher energy costs, and considerable increases in defense spending suggest an upcoming age of scarcity for education, urban, and social welfare constituencies. The specter of these needy and powerful interest groups doing battle for scarce federal dollars is not inviting, but it is a scenario that some analysts see as likely.

Not everyone believes that the "age of scarcity" scenario is inevitable. Jack Ossofsky (1978), Executive Director of the National Council on the Aging, takes exception to Samuelson's characterization of the federal budget as ready to bust, and to his calculations of aging expenditures in the federal budget. For example, Ossofsky points out that the social security program provides income to many younger men, women, and children as part of its dependents, survivors, and disability program. A U.S. Senate Special Committee on Aging (1980) report indicates that 16.1 million or almost 45 percent of the estimated 35.9 million beneficiaries of social security in 1981 are *not* retired workers but rather the disabled (2.9 million) and dependents and survivors (some of whom *are* aged). According to Ossofsky, almost one-third of all social security payments go to people under the age of sixty-five. In addition, we must remember that workers "buy in" to social security (as do their employers)—to include such contributions when computing government expenditures on behalf of the aged makes little sense. Beyond simply confusing matters, it creates the impression that social security is just another government "giveaway" rather than a return of money put aside during the course of a person's working years. This holds true as well for the Civil Service Retirement system, Military Retirement, and, until its recent integration into social security, the Railroad Retirement System. *Redistributed employee contributions should not be counted as government expenditures.* Actually, prior to 1969 these programs were excluded from presentations of the federal budget. Finally, Ossofsky argues that playing hocus pocus with the federal budget figures creates the false impression that the elderly are receiving lavish and extravagant treatment from the federal government. However, as we have already pointed out (See Chapter 2), 14 percent of America's aged have income below the poverty level and the proportion at risk for sinking below the poverty level is substantial as well.

Robert Butler (1978), first Director of the fledgling National Institute on Aging, takes a different approach. He suggests that the discussion of over expenditures on behalf of the aged in the federal budget is misdirected, a case of "blaming the victims." Butler makes three important points:

First, the need for all those dollars in retirement systems might be lessened somewhat if we did not pressure people to leave the work force while they are still able and willing to continue working. If people were free to continue working after age sixty-five or seventy—and they continued to contribute to retirement systems—the budget could become less problematic.

Second, a considerable proportion of the federal budget reflects the existence of illness and disability in the aged population. What if we could identify the biomedical (including nutritional) and socioenvironmental factors that contribute to illness and disability and prompt people to retire? A recent study of "very early retirees"—men who retire from work *before* age 62—shows that eighty percent of the black and 66 percent of the white very early retirees retired involuntarily. For the great majority of these men, poor health and disability are implicated in involuntary retirement (Special Committee on Aging, 1981). If these "illness factors" could be minimized in any way it would reduce expenditures made through Medicare and Medicaid.

Finally, government expenditures for health care services have increased dramatically in recent years. Nevertheless, the elderly now pay as much or more out-of-pocket for health care than before Medicare. Are the elderly to blame for this? To what extent is the increasing cost of health care and thus increasing government expenditures to be attributed to the providers of health care services?

Just what are the political consequences of a debate over federal expenditures for the elderly? Are programs for the aged to go without funding? Can the aged mobilize pressure to serve their interests? There is a commonly held image of the aged as a formidable political force capable of playing interest group politics. However, political scientist Robert Binstock, former president of the Gerontological Society of America, believes that this image is inaccurate, although it is reinforced by several organizations composed mainly of elderly members. According to Binstock (1978), whatever "senior power" exists is held by organizations that cannot swing decisive blocs of votes. Thus there is little reason to believe that such organizations will be able to hold their own or lobby for significant increases in the proportion of the budget devoted to the aging.

One reason for the persistence of the image of senior power lies in the belief that the elderly are a homogeneous political constituency. This belief would appear to be false. Binstock points out that most older voters do not identify themselves, and hence their self-interest, in terms of aging. When a person reaches age sixty-five, enters retirement status, or suffers widowhood, he or she does not suddenly lose all prior self-identities. Self-interest is still derived from factors of race, education, religion, and community ties, among other variables.

Do all agree that senior power is illusory? Pratt (1976) notes that the elderly have come to expect some degree of income security as well as adequate health care. Theirs may be a revolution of rising expectations. Pratt cites the 1971 White house Conference on Aging as the watershed for old-age political influence. Through the Conference, he argues, national groups such as the American Association of Retired Persons (AARP) and the National Council of Senior Citizens (NCSC) developed the political acumen necessary for effecting legislation that benefits the aged. Pratt credits the NCSC with helping to formulate and pass the Social Security Amendments of 1972. These amendments pegged increases in social security benefits to the rate of inflation and replaced welfare programs for the aged, blind, and disabled with SSI.

Can an old-age political movement become institutionalized and thus assure appropriate federal funding for health, nutrition, and other programs for the aged? Perhaps it can although much depends on the willingness of current and future generations of the elderly to identify themselves as old. The development of a widespread group consciousness among the aging would bring recognition among the elderly (and others) of their common interests. Bengtson and Cutler (1976) present evidence that older people who identify themselves as "old" are more liberal, particularly on issues affecting the aged, such as government intervention in inflation and medical care. The development of a group consciousness among older people may have important consequences beyond helping to create and sustain an old-age political movement. Not the least of these would be a lessening of the stigmatization and isolation of the aged and the maintenance of self-esteem.

SUMMARY

Systematic policies for dealing with dependent aged people began to be implemented in late sixteenth century England. One consequence of the Poor Laws was the development of so-called poorhouses, which were harsh and punitive environments that housed and fed the incapable and/or aged poor without families. American colonists followed the English model. By the latter part of the nineteenth century and early into the twentieth century a new attitude oriented toward caring for the aged emerged. This new attitude evolved into collective social action on behalf of the aged.

With the passage of the Social Security Act of 1935, the U.S. became one of the last industrial nations to establish a federal old-age pension program. Since then, though, chronological age has increasingly been used as the basis upon which to allocate the benefits of government programs. Contrary to much rhetoric about government neglect of the elderly, it would seem that the aged have become a favored social welfare constituency in the U.S.

Programs such as Food Stamps and Title III of the Older Americans Act are aimed specifically at maintaining or improving nutritional status. Social Security (including SSI), Medicare, and public housing programs have more indirect impact on nutritional status.

Some observers see the growing costs of federal programs for the elderly as the dominant factor shaping federal spending and taxing decisions in the coming years. Others argue that playing hocus pocus with the federal budget creates the false impression that the elderly are receiving extravagant treatment from the federal government.

STUDY QUESTIONS

1. What were the Poor Laws? What underlying social values helped shape these laws? How did these laws effect the development of specialty institutions for the elderly?

2. What changes in the socioeconomic and demographic structure of American society eventually led to the passage of the Social Security Act of 1935?

3. Distinguish between breakthrough and constituency-building policies. Which have had greater impact on the elderly in the U.S.? Are the aged a favored welfare constituency in the U.S.? Why do you think so?

4. What is the Food Stamp Program and how does it work? Why is it problematic to assume that receiving food stamps means an adequate diet is being provided?

5. How do the nutrition programs within the Older Americans Act seek to alleviate nutritional deficits of the elderly? Are these programs successful? Can you identify criticisms of the Title VII program? What are they?

6. What did the Social Security Act of 1935 establish for the first time in America? How is this program funded? What are its main effects on the elderly?

7. Discuss some socioeconomic and demographic circumstances that could effect the social security program now and in the future.

8. Describe the two basic components of the Medicare program. What does each one cover and how is each financed? Distinguish between Medicare and Medicaid.

9. Why do some fear that programs for the elderly may "bust the U.S. budget?" How may this fear be a case of "blaming the victims?"
10. Are the elderly a political force to be taken seriously? Or, is "senior power" illusory?

BIBLIOGRAPHY

ACHENBAUM, W. A., *Old Age in the New Land*. Baltimore, Md.: The Johns Hopkins University Press, 1978.

BENGTSON, V. and CUTLER, N., "Generations and Intergenerational Relations: Perspectives on Age Groups and Social Change," in *Handbook of Aging and the Social Sciences*, ed. by R. Binstock and E. Shanas. New York: Van Nostrand Reinhold, 1976.

BINSTOCK, R., "Federal Policy Toward the Aging—Its Inadequacies and Its Politics," *National Journal*, November 11 (1978), 1838–1845.

BOSKIN, M., *The Crisis in Social Security: Problems and Prospects*. San Francisco: Institute for Contemporary Studies, 1977.

BURGESS, E., *Aging in Western Societies*. Chicago: University of Chicago Press, 1960.

BUTLER, R., "The Economics of Aging: We Are Asking the Wrong Questions," *National Journal*, November 4 (1978), 1792–1797.

CALHOUN, R., *In Search of the New Old*. New York: Elsevier Scientific Publishing, 1978.

CARP, F., "Housing and the Living Environments of Older People," in *Handbook of Aging and the Social Sciences*, ed. by R. Binstock and E. Shanas. New York: Van Nostrand Reinhold, 1976.

CROCKER, J. C., *A Brief History of Old Age Institutions in the U.S.* (mimeographed). Charlottesville, Va.: Center for Program Effectiveness Studies, 1974.

ESTES, C., *The Aging Enterprise*. San Francisco: Jossey-Bass, 1979.

FISCHER, D., *Growing Old in America*. New York: Oxford University Press, 1977.

FOX, A., "Earnings Replacement Rates of Retired Couples: Findings From the Retirement History Study," *Social Security Bulletin*, January (1979), 17–39.

GOLD, B., KUTZA, E., MARMOR, T., "United States Social Policy on Old Age: Present Patterns and Predictions," in *Social Policy, Social Ethics, and the Aging Society*, ed. by B. Neugarten and R. Havighurst. Washington, D.C.: National Science Foundation, 1977.

HOLLISTER, R., "Social Mythology and Reform: Income Maintenance for the Aged," *Annals of the American Academy of Political and Social Sciences*, 415 (1974), 19–40.

HUDSON, R., "The 'Graying' of the Federal Budget and Its Consequences for Old-Age Policy," *Gerontologist*, 18 (1978), 428–439.

KART, C., *The Realities of Aging*. Boston: Allyn and Bacon, 1981.

KELSO, R., *History of Poor Relief in Massachusetts*. Boston: Houghton Mifflin & Company, 1922.

KUTZA, E. A., *The Benefits of Old Age*. Chicago: University of Chicago Press, 1981.

LAKOFF, S. A., "The Future of Social Intervention," in *Handbook of Aging and the Social Sciences*, ed. by R. Binstock and E. Shanas. New York: Van Nostrand Reinhold, 1976.

LAWTON, M. P., *Environment and Aging*. Monterey, California: Brooks/Cole, 1980.

MACDONALD, M., *Food Stamps, and Income Maintenance*. New York: Academic Press, 1977.

MACFARLANE, A., *Witchcraft in Tudor and Stuart England*. London: Routledge & Kegan Paul, 1970.

MADDOX, G. and WILEY, J., "Scope, Concepts and Methods in the Study of Aging," in *Handbook of Aging and the Social Sciences*, eds. R. Binstock and E. Shanas. New York: Van Nostrand Reinhold, 1976.

MANARD, B., KART, C. S., and VAN GILS, D., *Old Age Institutions*. Lexington, Massachusetts: Heath, 1975.

MARMOR, T., *The Politics of Medicare*. Chicago: Aldine, 1973.

MEENAGHAN, T. M. and WASHINGTON, R. O., *Social Policy and Social Welfare*. New York: Free Press, 1980.

MENCHER, S., *Poor Law to Poverty Programs*. Pittsburgh: University of Pittsburgh Press, 1967.

MUNNELL, A., *The Future of Social Security*. Washington, D.C.: The Brookings Institution, 1977.

OSSOFSKY, J., "Through the Aging Budget—One More Time," *National Journal*, March 11 (1978), 408–409.

POSNER, B. M., *Nutrition and the Elderly*. Lexington, Mass.: D.C. Heath, Lexington Books, 1979.

PRATT, H., *The Gray Lobby*. Chicago: University of Chicago Press, 1976.

PUTNAM, J. K., *Old-Age Politics in California: From Richardson to Reagan*. Stanford, Calif.: Stanford University Press, 1970.

SAMUELSON, R., "Busting the U.S. Budget—The Costs of an Aging America," *National Journal*, February 18 (1978), 256–260.

SCHMANDT, J., SHOREY, R., and KINCH, L., *Nutrition Policy in Transition*. Lexington, Mass.: D.C. Heath, Lexington Books, 1980.

SEXAUER, B., "The U.S. Food Stamp Programme," *Food Policy*, November (1977), 331–337.

Special Committee on Aging, U.S. Senate, *Developments in Aging: 1978 (Part I)*. Washington, D.C.: U.S. Government Printing Office, 1979.

Special Committee on Aging, U.S. Senate, *The Proposed Fiscal 1981 Budget: What It Means for Older Americans*. Washington, D.C.: U.S. Government Printing Office, 1980.

Special Committee on Aging, U.S. Senate, *The Myth of Early Retirement*. Washington, D.C.: U.S. Government Printing Office, 1981.

STEVENS, R. and STEVENS, R., *Welfare Medicine in America: A Case Study of Medicaid*. New York: Free Press, 1974.

TRATTNER, W. I., *From Poor Law to Welfare State* (Second Edition). New York: Free Press, 1979.

U.S. Department of Agriculture, Food and Nutrition Services, *Characteristics of Food Stamp Households: September, 1976*. Washington, D.C.: U.S. Government Printing Office, 1977.

U.S. Department of Health, Education, and Welfare, *The Measure of Poverty—Food Plans for Poverty Measurement*. Washington, D.C.: U.S. Government Printing Office, 1976.

U.S. Department of Housing and Urban Development, *Housing for the Elderly and Handicapped*. Washington, D.C.: Office of Policy Development and Research, USHUD, 1979.

U.S. Senate Committee on Finance, *The Supplementary Security Income Program*. Washington, D.C.: U.S. Government Printing Office, 1977.

WATKIN, D., "The Nutrition Program for Older Americans: A Successful Application of Current Knowledge in Nutrition and Gerontology," *World Review of Nutrition and Diet.*, 26 (1977), 26.

EPILOGUE
TOWARD A NATIONAL
NUTRITION POLICY?

The National Nutrition Consortium developed five general goals to be addressed by a national nutrition policy (Select Committee on Nutrition and Human Needs, 1974a). These are as follows:

1. Assure an adequate wholesome food supply at reasonable cost to meet the needs of all segments of the population. This supply is to be available at a level consistent with the affordable lifestyle of the era.
2. Maintain food resources sufficient to meet emergency needs, and fulfill a responsible role as a nation in meeting world food needs.
3. Develop a level of sound public knowledge and responsible understanding of nutrition and foods that will promote maximal nutritional knowledge.
4. Maintain a system of quality and safety control that justifies public confidence in its food supply.
5. Support research and education in foods and nutrition with adequate resources and reasoned priorities to solve important current problems and to permit exploratory basic research.

These goals have been described as abstract, but even if they were presented with greater specification (for the general population or the elderly), could they be implemented? The answer would seem to be no. The 1969 White House Conference on Nutrition Report stated that "Balkanization of responsibilities and authorities constitute a serious barrier to a concerted attack on hunger and malnutrition." Government organization for the implementation of nutritional goals would seem to be only modestly better today than it was in 1969. This is the case in spite of the eight organizational proposals of the 1969 White House Conference.

1. Federal machinery for food and nutrition be administered as a total system under clear policy guidance, accountability, program management, and independent evaluation.

2. A special assistant to the President be designated to follow through on the Conference recommendations and serve as eyes and ears for the President.

3. The Secretary of DHEW be assigned Executive Order responsibilities for government-wide policy and coordination.

4. Establish at a high level in DHEW an Office of Nutrition to formulate and carry through policy priorities of DHEW.

5. The Assistant Secretary of DHEW for Health and Medical Affairs to plan and implement an effective nutrition surveillance and monitoring system linked to state, county, and local units.

6. That DHEW plan and carry out nutrition surveillance and monitoring aimed at selected target populations and areas.

7. USDA's family, household, and individual food surveys coordinated with nutrition and health surveillance and placed on a five-year schedule.

8. That state and local public health agencies be supplemented by Area Nutrition Service Centers funded by DHEW.

A 1974 report of the Panel on Nutrition and Government of the U.S. Senate Select Committee on Nutrition and Human Needs offers three reasons for the lack of action on a national nutrition policy. First, it would seem that nutrition is a low federal priority. In 1973, the President directed every major department and agency to define its high-priority objectives. Early in 1974, 144 Federal objectives received presidential approval. Two of these were concerned with nutrition: (1) the "development of a cost-effective child nutrition program," and (2) the "rationalization of eligibility requirements for food stamps." Nutrition will continue to be a low-priority item for the federal government as long as it fails to make the distinction between hunger and nutrition. As the above-mentioned report indicates, hunger has indeed been alleviated in America, but the goal of improved nutrition has not made the same headway.

Second, the preeminent policy viewpoint in the federal government seems to associate nutrition with "income maintenance" programs rather than with health policies. For example, the 1975 presidential budget message proposed the "transfer of food stamps and related nutrition programs to the Department of HEW to improve coordination of income maintenance programs." This emphasis on income maintenance continues. Until cutbacks by the Reagan administration, the Food Stamp Program had expanded to reach the poor and working poor who were not eligible for othe forms of income support.

Finally, the poor quality of the government's information on the status of nutrition and health probably precludes any breakthrough in national nutrition policy. It is fragmentary, partial, improvised, and unreliable (Select Committee on Nutrition and Human Needs, 1974b). In part, this is because no single focus exists in the executive branch of government to assess and advocate nutrition policies.

A fourth reason (not developed by the Senate Select Committee) for the lack of action on a national nutrition policy has to do with the difficulty of achieving consensus among nutrition experts about public policy issues. A consideration of the proposed dietary goals for the United States should exemplify this problem.

DIETARY GOALS

In 1977, the U.S. Senate Select Committee on Nutrition and Human Needs proposed a set of dietary goals for the United States (See Table 8.1). The goals were not to be viewed as a panacea for disease, but rather as healthful guides to follow. In part they represent an outgrowth of concern that dietary changes occurring in the U.S. since the beginning of this century pose a significant threat to the nation's health. While the Committee recognized the continued existence of malnutrition, it argued that the major dietary concern for the United States as a whole is the problem of "over-nutrition"—eating too much of the wrong foods. In an introduction to the *Dietary Goals*, it is noted that six of the ten leading causes of death in the United States have been linked to our diet. These include heart disease, stroke and cancer, and conditions that appear to be related to lifestyle factors such as diet (see Chapter 6). The goals

TABLE 8.1.   U.S. dietary goals, 1977.

1. To avoid overweight, consume only as much energy as is expended; if overweight, decrease energy intake and increase energy expenditure.
2. Increase the consumption of complex carbohydrates and "naturally ocurring" sugars from about 28 percent of energy intake to about 48 percent of energy intake.
3. Reduce the consumption of refined and processed sugars by about 45 percent to account for about 10 percent of total energy intake.
4. Reduce overall fat consumption from approximately 40 percent to about 30 percent of energy intake.
5. Reduce saturated fat consumption to account for about 10 percent of total energy intake, and balance that with polyunsaturated and monounsaturated fats, which should account for about 10 percent of energy intake each.
6. Reduce cholesterol consumption to about 300 mg./day.
7. Limit the intake of sodium by reducing the intake of salt to about 5 gm./day.

Source: U.S. Senate Select Committee on Nutrition and Human Needs. *Dietary Goals for the United States, Revised Edition.* Washington, D.C.: U.S. Government Printing Office, 1977.

were endorsed by a number of prominent nutrition and health authorities. In Senate testimony, the noted nutritionist D. M. Hegsted emphasized:

> The diet we eat today was not planned or developed for any particular purpose. It is a happenstance related to our affluence, the productivity of our farmers and the activities of our food industry. The risks associated with eating this diet are demonstrably large. The question to be asked, therefore, is not why should we change our diet, but why not? What are the risks associated with less salt, and more fruits, vegetables, unsaturated fat and cereal products—especially whole grain cereals? There are none that can be identified and important benefits can be expected.

Despite these endorsements, there has been considerable controversy over the goals. One concern involved the state of scientific evidence on the relationship between nutrition and disease. Some believe the evidence to be sufficiently incomplete to make recommendations to the public contraindicated. An emphasis on the goals without any significant improvement in the incidence of disease might undermine confidence in professional advice concerning health habits. More specifically, nutrition science might suffer if future research indicated the need for a *new* set of dietary goals. Later advice might also be ignored if the stated goals appeared unjustifiable.

The concerns of some critics were clearly a consequence of economic considerations. As Caliendo (1981) has pointed out, the institutionalization of the goals could have drastic economic repercussions. If the demand for food shifts from animal and dairy products to more fresh produce and whole-grain products, there could be severe economic problems for the dairy and meat sectors. Would we change agricultural policies and provide price supports to improve the income of producers of grain, fruits, and vegetables rather than the producers of meat, egg, and dairy products?

In 1980, the Departments of Agriculture and Health, Education and Welfare reacted to the controversy over the goals by publishing the more general set of dietary guidelines listed below.

1. Eat a variety of foods daily.
2. Maintain ideal weight.
3. Avoid too much fat, unsaturated fat, and cholesterol.
4. Eat foods with adequate starch and fiber.
5. Avoid too much sugar.
6. Avoid too much sodium.
7. If you drink alcohol, do so in moderation.

But even here, the controversy did not die. Later in 1980, the Food and Nutrition Board of the National Academy of Sciences published a report entitled *Toward Healthful Diets*. This report deviated from the dietary guidelines listed above in the areas of fat, cholesterol, and carbohydrates in the diet. For example, the Food and Nutrition Board said that only people at risk for heart disease should worry about cholesterol. They remarked that only obese individuals and those at risk of heart disease should be concerned about fat and that only diabetics should be concerned about fat and the mix of sugars and complex carbohydrates (Hitt, 1982). Interestingly, both sets of guidelines were based on an examination of the same scientific evidence. What accounts for the differences in recommendations? Hitt (1982) suggests an explanation. He argues that whereas the government looked at the total population and what could be done to improve the health of people in general, the Food and Nutrition Board seems to have approached the matter clinically, as a physician would treat a single patient.

The incompleteness of scientific evidence on the relationship between nutrition and health and the lack of consensus as to what constitutes appropriate dietary goals (or guidelines, for that matter) for the U.S. population would seem to indicate that formulation of a national nutrition policy is a very remote possibility. The currently popular political ideology that views federal involvement in social and health programs in negative terms is also strong evidence that the likelihood of such a policy is still only a dim vision of some possible future.

BIBLIOGRAPHY

CALINEDO, M., *Nutrition and Preventive Health Care.* New York: Macmillian, 1981.
Food and Nutrition Board, *Toward Healthful Diets.* Washington, D.C.: National Academy of Sciences, 1980.
HITT, C., "Risk Reduction: A Community Strategy," *Community Nutritionist,* January-February (1982), 12–17.
Select Committee on Nutrition and Human Needs, *Guidelines for a National Nutrition Policy.* Washington, D.C.: U.S. Government Printing Office, 1974a.
————, *National Nutrition Policy Study, Report and Recommendations—II.* Washington, D.C.: U.S. Government Printing Office, 1974b.

APPENDIX I
INFORMATION SOURCES IN GERIATRIC NUTRITION

I. Abstracting services
   A. Nutrition Abstracts and Reviews
   B. Biological Abstracts
   C. Excerpta Medica: Gerontology and Geriatrics
   D. Excerpta Medica: Public Health and Hygiene
   E. Research and Abstracts for Social Workers
   F. Human Resources Abstracts

II. Indexing services
   A. Bibliography of Agriculture
   B. Bioresearch Index
   C. Index Medicus
   D. Monthly Catalog of United States Government Publications
   E. Public Affairs Information Services
   F. Social Science Index
   G. Human and Animal Aging: Bioresearch Today

III. Nutrition journals with information on geriatric nutrition
   A. *American Journal Clinical Nutrition*
   B. *British Journal of Nutrition*
   C. *Canadian Nutrition and Notes*
   D. *Community Nutritionist*
   E. *Diabetes*
   F. *Diabetes Educator*
   G. *Food and Nutrition Notes*
   H. *Human Ecology Forum*

I. *Journal of the American College of Nutrition*
J. *Journal of the American Dietetic Association*
K. *Journal of the Canadian Dietetic Association*
L. *Journal of Home Economics*
M. *Journal of Human Nutrition*
N. *Journal of Nutrition Education*
O. *Journal of Nutrition for the Elderly*
P. *Nutrition Reviews*
Q. *Nutrition Today*
R. *Proceedings of the Nutrition Society*
S. *Progress in Food and Nutrition*

IV. Gerontology journals that carry articles on nutrition
   A. *Age and Aging*
   B. *British Journal of Geriatric Practice*
   C. *Geriatrics*
   D. *Gerontology* (formerly *Gerontological* and *Gerontologia Clinica*)
   E. *Journal of the American Geriatrics Society*
   F. *Journal of Gerontology*
   G. *The Gerontologist*
   H. *Journal of Gerontological Nursing*
   I. *Geriatric Nursing*
   J. *Archives in Gerontology and Geriatrics*

V. Miscellaneous publications that carry articles on nutrition related to the elderly
   A. *Community Nutrition Institute Weekly Report*
   B. *Annual Review of Nutrition*
   C. *World Review of Nutrition and Dietetics*

VI. Bibliographies
   A. Metress, S. P. and C. S. Kart. 1979. Nutrition and Aging: Bibliographic Survey. Public Administration Series, p. 309. Vance Bibliographies, Monticello, Illinois
   B. Weg, R. B. 1977. Nutrition and Aging: A Selected Bibliography. Technical Bibliographies on Aging. Andrus Gerontological Center. University of Southern California. Los Angeles.
   C. Society for Nutrition Education. 1976. Aging and Nutrition. Nutrition Education Resource Series No. 5, SNE, Berkeley, California.
   D. Shock, N. 1946–1980. Current Publications in Gerontology and Geriatrics in the *Journal of Gerontology* (subsections on nutrition).
   E. Simko, M. D. and K. S. Babich. 1974. Home Delivered Meals: A Selected Annotated Bibliography. Dept. Health, Education, and Welfare, Washington, D. C.
   F. Simko, M. D. and K. Colitz. 1973. Nutrition and Aging: A Selected Annotated Bibliography, 1964-1972. Dept. Health, Education and Welfare, Washington, D. C.
   G. National Library of Medicine. 1981. Nutrition and the Elderly. January 1977 through 1981. Library of Medicine, Bethesda, Maryland.

APPENDIX II

TABLE 1 Recommended daily dietary allowances,[a] Revised 1980. Designed for the maintenance of good nutrition of practically all healthy people in the U.S.A.

	Age (years)	Weight (kg)	Weight (lb)	Height (cm)	Height (in)	Protein (g)	FAT-SOLUBLE VITAMINS Vitamin A (μg RE)[b]	FAT-SOLUBLE VITAMINS Vitamin D (μg)[c]	FAT-SOLUBLE VITAMINS Vitamin E (mg α-TE)[d]	WATER-SOLUBLE VITAMINS Vitamin C (mg)	WATER-SOLUBLE VITAMINS Thiamin (mg)
Infants	0.0-0.5	6	13	60	24	kg × 2.2	420	10	3	35	0.3
	0.05-1.0	9	20	71	28	kg × 2.0	400	10	4	35	0.5
Children	1-3	13	29	90	35	23	400	10	5	45	0.7
	4-6	20	44	112	44	30	500	10	6	45	0.9
	7-10	28	62	132	52	34	700	10	7	45	1.2
Males	11-14	45	99	157	62	45	1000	10	8	50	1.4
	15-18	66	145	176	69	56	1000	10	10	60	1.4
	19-22	70	154	177	70	56	1000	7.5	10	60	1.5
	23-50	70	154	178	70	56	1000	5	10	60	1.4
	51+	70	154	178	70	56	1000	5	10	60	1.2
Females	11-14	46	101	157	62	46	800	10	8	50	1.1
	15-18	55	120	163	64	46	800	10	8	60	1.1
	19-22	55	120	163	64	44	800	7.5	8	60	1.1
	23-50	55	120	163	64	44	800	5	8	60	1.0
	51+	55	120	163	64	44	800	5	8	60	1.0
Pregnant						+30	+200	+5	+2	+20	+0.4
Lactating						+20	+400	+5	+3	+40	+0.5

[a] The allowances are intended to provide for individual variations among most normal persons as they live in the United States under usual environmental stresses. Diets should be based on a variety of common foods in order to provide other nutrients for which human requirements have been less well defined.

[b] Retinol equivalents. 1 retinol equivalent = μg retinol or 6 μg β carotene. See text for calculation of vitamin A activity of diets as retinol equivalents.

[c] As cholecalciferol. 10μg cholecalciferol = 400 IU of vitamin D.

[d] α-tocopherol equivalents. 1 mg d-α tocopherol = 1 α-TE. See text for variation in allowances and calculation of vitamin E activity of the diet as α-tocopherol equivalents.

[e] 1 NE(niacin equivalent) is equal to 1 mg of niacin or 60 mg of dietary tryptophan.

[f] The folacin allowances refer to dietary sources as determined by *Lactobacillus casei* assay after treatment with enzymes (conjugases) to make polyglutamyl forms of the vitamin available to the test organism.

WATER-SOLUBLE VITAMINS					MINERALS					
Ribo-flavin (mg)	Niacin (mg NE)	Vita-min B-6 (mg)	Fola-cin^f (µg)	Vitamin B-12 (µg)	Cal-cium (mg)	Phos-phorus (mg)	Mag-nesium (mg)	Iron (mg)	Zinc (mg)	Iodine (µg)
0.4	6	0.3	30	0.5^a	360	240	50	10	3	40
0.6	8	0.6	45	1.5	540	360	70	15	5	50
0.8	9	0.9	100	2.0	800	800	150	15	10	70
1.0	11	1.3	200	2.5	800	800	200	10	10	90
1.4	16	1.6	300	3.0	800	800	250	10	10	120
1.6	18	1.8	400	3.0	1200	1200	350	18	15	150
1.7	18	2.0	400	3.0	1200	1200	400	18	15	150
1.7	19	2.2	400	3.0	800	800	350	10	15	150
1.6	18	2.2	400	3.0	800	800	350	10	15	150
1.4	16	2.2	400	3.0	800	800	350	10	15	150
1.3	15	1.8	400	3.0	1200	1200	300	18	15	150
1.3	14	2.0	400	3.0	1200	1200	300	18	15	150
1.3	14	2.0	400	3.0	800	800	300	18	15	150
1.2	13	2.0	400	3.0	800	800	300	18	15	150
1.2	13	2.0	400	3.0	800	800	300	10	15	150
+ 0.3	+ 2	+ 0.6	+ 400	+ 1.0	+ 400	+ 400	+ 150	h	+ 5	+ 25
+ 0.5	+ 5	+ 0.5	+ 100	+ 1.0	+ 400	+ 400	+ 150	h	+ 10	+ 50

g The recommended dietary allowance for vitamin B-12 in infants is based on average concentration of the vitamin in human milk. The allowances after weaning are based on energy intake (as recommended by the American Academy of Pediatrics) and consideration of other factors, such as intestinal absorption.

h The increased requirement during pregnancy cannot be met by the iron content of habitual American diets nor by the existing iron stores of many women; therefore the use of 30-60 mg of supplemental iron is recommended. Iron needs during lactation are not substantially different from those of nonpregnant women, but continued supplementation of the mother for 2-3 months after parturition is advisable in order to replenish stores depleted by pregnancy.

Food and Nutrition Board, National Academy of Sciences—National Research Council, Washington, D.C.

GLOSSARY

Abkhasians   The long-lived people of the Soviet state of Georgia; they attribute their
    longevity to practices in sex, work, and diet.

acute illness   A condition, disease, or disorder that is temporary.

adipose   Referring to fat tissue.

age-specific life expectancy   The average duration of life expected for an individual of
    a given stated age.

amino acids   The structural components of protein.

antedeluvian theme   Involves the belief that people lived much longer in the past.

antioxidant   A substance that prevents or retards oxidation.

arteriosclerosis   A generic term indicating a hardening of or loss of elasticity of the
    arteries.

arthritis   Inflammation and/or degenerative joint change often characterized by
    stiffening, swelling, and joint pain.

ascorbic acid   Vitamin C.

atherosclerosis   A condition whereby the tunica intima or inner wall of an artery
    becomes thickened by plaque formation.

autoimmune theory   This theory maintains that because of "copying errors" in
    repeated cell divisions, protein enzymes produced by newer cells are literally not
    recognized by the body. This brings the body's immunologic system into play,
    forcing it to work against itself.

baby boom   Often used to describe the higher fertility rates in the years immediately
    following World War II.

Bacteroides   A genus of bacteria.

basal metabolism rate (BMR)   The total energy output of the body at rest after a 12-
    hour fast.

biotin   A B-complex vitamin.

calculus   Deposits of tartar on the teeth.

cataract   An opacity of the lens of the eye.

cerebrovascular disease   Used to describe impaired brain cell circulation. When a portion of the brain is completely denied of blood, a cerebrovascular accident or stroke occurs.

cholecystitis   Inflammation of the gall bladder.

chronic illness   A condition, disease, or disorder that is permanent or that will incapacitate an individual for a long period of time.

cirrhosis of liver   Hardening of liver tissue.

Clostridia   A genus of bacteria.

coenzyme   A small molecule that works with an enzyme to promote the enzyme's activity.

collagen   A supportive protein of connective tissue.

corticosteroid   A compound, derived from the adrenal cortex or a compound prepared synthetically with a similar structure.

decubitus ulcer   Pressure sores, also known as bedsores.

degenerative disease   The deterioration in the structure or function of cells, tissues, or organs in disease.

demography   The study of the size, territorial distribution and composition of population, and the changes therein.

dental caries   Tooth decay.

diabetes mellitus   A metabolic disorder in which the body does not properly utilize carbohydrates.

diuretics   Agents that induce the flow of urine.

diverticulosis   Outpouching of the wall of an organ, usually the intestine.

dopamine   An intermediate product in the synthesis of morepinephrine.

endentulousness   Without teeth.

epithelial tissue   A type of connection tissue that covers the body.

familial dependency ratio   Defined in simple demographic terms (for example, population 65–79/population 45–49), this ratio crudely illustrates the shifts in the ratio of elderly parents to the children who would support them.

fertility rate   The number of births that occur in a year per 1,000 women of child-bearing age.

fibroblasts   Embryonic cells which give rise to connective tissue.

folacin   Folic acid, a B-complex vitamin.

fountain theme   Based on the idea that there is some unusual substance which has the property of greatly increasing the length of life.

gerontology   The systematic study of the aging process.

gingivitis   Inflammation of the gums.

glomerulonephritis   Inflammation of the glomeruli of the kidneys.

glucose   A simple sugar sometimes known as blood sugar.

glycosuria   The presence of abnormal sugar in the urine.

gout   An inherited condition of abnormal purine metabolism characterized by excess levels of uric acid.

hematocrit   The volume percentage of red blood cells in whole blood.

hemmorrhoids   Varicose veins in the walls of the anus.

hemodialysis   Artificially cleansing the blood.

hemoglobin   A blood protein that is necessary for oxygen exchange in the cells and tissues.

hepato-biliary tract   Pertaining to the liver and gall bladder.

hiatus hernia   Protrusion of any structure through the esophageal hiatus of the diaphragm.

hyperborean theme   Involves the idea that in some remote part of the world there are people who enjoy a remarkably long life.

hypercholesteremia   Too much cholesterol.

hyperparathyroidism   Overactive parathyroid gland.

hypertension   High blood pressure.

hypervitaminoses   Vitamin poisoning due to excess ingestion.

hypogastric   Reduced secretary activity of the stomach.

hypoglycemia   Low blood sugar.

keratinization   The filling and thickening of epithetial cells with keratin.

lactase deficiency   A deficiency of the enzyme lactase which is necessary for the digestion of lactose, a major component of milk and other dairy products.

L-dopa   A drug used to control the symptoms of Parkinson's disease.

life span   The extreme limit of human longevity, the age beyond which no one can expect to live.

life table   Shows what the probability is of surviving from any age to any subsequent age based on the death rates at a particular time and place.

lipoproteins   A complex of lipids with proteins which have been implicated in heart disease.

lysine   One of the body's essential amino acids.

lysosomes   Saclike structures in the cell cytoplasm containing digestive enzymes which implement the breakdown of fats, proteins, and nucleic acids. Lysosomes have been implicated in cellular aging.

malabsorption syndromes   A variety of functional conditions that are characterized by poor absorption of nutrients in the G. I. tract.

malignant neoplasms   Cancer.

mandibular dentures   Lower dental plates.

maxillary dentures   Upper dental plates.

Medicaid   A public program for indigent persons of all ages paid for with matching federal and state funds. Medicaid has become the principal public mechanism for funding nursing home care.

Medicare   A federal insurance program financing a portion of the health-care costs of persons aged sixty-five and over.

megadose   Intake of a nutrient in a quantity larger than is considered normal.

methionine   One of the body's essential amino acids.

morbidity   The condition of being ill; often used to refer to the rate of illness per unit of population in a society.

mortality rate   The total number of deaths in a year per 1,000 individuals in the society.

neurons   Nerve cells.

niacin   A B-complex vitamin also known as nicotinic acid.

nutrition   The science that deals with the effects of food on the body.

obesity   Excessive body fatness generally defined as 15 to 20 percent overweight.

old-age dependency ratio   The ratio of the population too old to work to the population of working age.

"old-old"   Those persons seventy-five years of age and older.

organic brain syndrome   A constellation of psychological or behavior signs and symptoms without references to etiology.

osteoarthritis   Also known as degenerative joint disease, characterized by chronic breakdown of joint tissue.

osteomalacia   Adult equivalent of rickets or vitamin D deficiency.

osteoporosis   Demineralization of bone, often associated with aging.

pancreatic lipase   A fat-digesting enzyme produced by the pancreas.

pantothenic acid   A B-complex vitamin.

parenteral   Generally referring to medications given through a route other than the mouth.

Parkinson's disease   A central nervous system condition.

periodontal disease   Pathological condition involving the main membrane surrounding the teeth.

pernicious anemia   A nutritional blood deficiency due to lack of vitamin B_{12}.

plaque   An accumulation of material on the teeth; also an accumulation of lipid material mixed with smooth muscle cells and calcium which is lodged in the artery walls.

polyunsaturated fats (PUFA)   Fats composed of triglycerides containing a high percentage of polyunsaturated fatty acids, implicated by some in the development of heart disease.

Poor Laws   Relief for the poor, passed during the reign of Elizabeth I.

poverty index   Developed by the Social Security Administration and based on the amount of money needed to purchase a minimum adequate diet as determined by the Department of Agriculture; it is the most frequently used measure of income adequacy.

prolongevity   Used to describe attempts to significantly extend the length of the human life span.

prothrombin   A blood protein necessary for blood clotting.

pyridoxine   Vitamin B_6, a B-complex vitamin.

R.D.A.   Recommended daily allowance, in reference to nutrient needs.

retirement test   A "test" employed by the Social Security Administration to determine whether or not a person otherwise eligible for retirement benefits can be considered retired.

rheumatoid arthritis   A major form of arthritis, characterized by crippling and disability.

riboflavin   Vitamin B_2, a B-complex vitamin.

senescence   Used by biological gerontologists to describe all the postmaturational changes in an individual.

sex ratio   The number of males for every 100 females (x 100).

sigmoid colon   That lower part of the large intestine shaped like the letter S.

social gerontology   The study of the impact of social and sociocultural factors on the aging process.

social security   The colloquial term used to describe the Old Age Survivors, Disability, and Health Insurance (OASDHI) program administered by the federal government. The most well-known aspect of this program is the public retirement pension system which provides income support to over 90 percent of American elderly.

Supplemental Security Income   (SSI) A Federal assistance program envisioned to supplement the existing incomes of eligible aged to bring them up to a minimal income level.

tissue necrosis   A death of tissue.

thiamine   Vitamin B_1, a B-complex vitamin.

tooth hydroxyapatite   The major calcium-containing crystal of bones and teeth.

transferrin   The body's iron-carrying protein.

triangulation   A research strategy that involves the use of multiple measurement techniques.

tryptophan   One of the ten essential amino acids or protein building blocks.

vascular tissue   Blood vessels.

Veillonella   A genus of bacteria.

wear-and-tear theory of aging Theorists using this biological model of aging often employ machine analogies to exemplify the theory's underlying assumption that an organism wears out with use or stress.

"young-old" Those persons aged fifty-five to seventy-four years.

Index